Effect of Meditation on Cardiovascular Health, Immunity & Brain Fitness

Effect of Meditation on Cardiovascular Health, Immunity & Brain Fitness

By

Annie Wilson

.

INNER LIGHT PUBLISHERS
www.inner-light-in.com

Table of Contents

Preface

Meditation has grown to a discipline that had previously been practiced only for the purpose of general wellbeing to something that is widely researched in modern research laboratories as a disease control and prevention therapy. Basic research in meditation has expanded enormously during the past two decades. We now possess an arsenal of scientifically proven and effective meditation techniques that are used for curing and preventing a wide spectrum of diseases as diverse as anxiety disorder, depression, or arthritis to cardiovascular diseases and Alzheimer's. This book is intended to serve as a simplified bridge between meditation practitioners, meditation researchers and the physicians. The original motivation for writing this book was the need for such a text voiced by physicians.

The chapters are designed and edited to read in sequence but are sufficiently cross-referenced so that they can be used out of order. Emphasis has been placed to understand the relation between meditation and cardiovascular health and brain fitness.

This book would not have happened without the help of many people that extended their helping hands in a most generous way. I am grateful to all of them. It has been a great privilege for me to collaborate with talented and creative medical students and physicians who helped me a lot in documenting the current research trends. Finally, a project of this magnitude could not be completed without the support of my family, and for that I am grateful to my parents, my husband Peter and my two daughters Isabella and Irene.

I hope that this book will enhance your understanding about scientific aspect of meditation. This book will provide a solid foundation for further learning on the effect of meditation on health and clinical care through meditation.

Introduction

One of the most interesting aspects of meditation research is to understand the impact of various meditation techniques for curing diseases. Whenever I talk on the subject of meditation, I found that people are more curious on the topic when I explain how the techniques can contribute to improve their physical health and mental wellbeing. This is understandable. Meditation had long been thought as an esoteric discipline that grants spiritual experiences, and ultimately enlightenment or self-realization, which has little relevance in our daily life. In modern high paced life, most of us need to do our jobs, interact with people, keep ourselves fit and take care of our loved ones. Here where does meditation fit in, if it doesn't give us some tangible benefits? That is true. Though meditation can lead us to freedom from sorrow, it also provides some immediate tangible benefits in the form of better physical and mental health. Even if you practice meditation for what I term as 'the by-products', you'll not be deprived of the benefits that it brings inevitably in the long run.

You know, only some twenty to thirty years before, it would sound such a strange, almost bizarre, even ridiculous idea to talk on meditation at a venue like a hospital or nursing home, because, three to four decades ago, meditation and medication or healthcare were supposed to be two absolutely unrelated disciplines. Why? Because, one was thought to be some other worldly activity, having little or no practical use, and other, a very necessary practical thing - related to our everyday life. Meditation was thought to have no practical uses- It was highly dogmatized and was associated with gurus, temples, worship and such so called 'spiritual' or abstruse things.

But things have changed since them, and with a growing body of scientific research coming out to back it, meditation has been an interesting subject from the angle of physical and mental health and well being. In many hospitals and universities across the world, meditation is being introduced as an alternative intervention and doctors are experimenting with clinical application of meditation to treat their patients.

Now there are over 3,000 scientific studies on the benefits of meditation. The therapeutic benefit of meditation on the physical and mental health of the individual has been unquestionably proven. In this book, I have discussed the impact of meditation on physical and mental health, with special reference to cardiovascular and brain fitness.

Cardiovascular health is a term used to describe health of the heart and the blood vessels. Cardiovascular health declines with smoking, chronic inflammation, high blood pressure, high blood cholesterol, too little or too much physical activity, stress, worry, overweight, obesity, poor nutrition and diabetes. Major cardiovascular diseases are: coronary heart disease, stroke, heart failure and peripheral vascular disease. Cardiovascular health improves with healthy eating and healthy lifestyle and meditation.

There is a growing body of research to back the claim that meditation can be used to prevent, even cure cardiovascular diseases as well as improve brain fitness.

Brain fitness is the ability of a human being to meet efficiently the diverse cognitive demands of everyday life. It includes the ability to assimilate information, understand relationships, and develop reasonable conclusions and plans. Scientific research confirmed that meditation along with sound sleep, healthy lifestyle, mental stimulation, physical exercise and good nutrition can improve brain fitness. On the other hand, chronic stress, anxiety and depression can decrease brain fitness. Chronic stress increases the stress hormone cortisol and adversely affects many brain functions. The stress hormone Cortisol creates a surplus of the neurotransmitter glutamate, which generates free radicals, unattached oxygen molecules that attack brain cells punching holes in the brain cell walls, causing the cells to rupture and die. Memory problems may be one of the first signs of stress you'll notice. For centuries meditation has been known as a great buster that also improves brain fitness and mind power. In this book we'll find that modern research strongly validates this claim.

Truly speaking, the benefits of meditation affect four dimensions of our being: physical, mental, emotional, and spiritual. The scope of this book is confined only to the first two aspects, because medical science considers health as 'absence of diseases'. But is health truly just absence of diseases?

A so-called healthy disease-free person — disease-free, in terms of physical and mental health diagnosable through instrument based evidences — may live a life full of absolute emotional turbulence. Can we not infer that the person is unhealthy emotionally? Emotional turbulence and destructive mental states like anxiety, anger, fear, hatred, resentment or worry, if continue for long, can manifest in diseases at the level of body or mind in the long run, though today a person may look perfectly healthy so far as the medical instruments diagnose. While exploring the body-mind connection, medical researchers have linked certain illnesses to our state of mind and emotional condition. They found that when you undergo mental stress, emotional pain, or depression, your physical resistance to disease drops.

Health, in true sense, is a state of wholeness, which is a feeling of perfect wellness. Health is not just confined to the body and the mind but it is also connected with the consciousness. To attain a perfect state of health, one has to remain mentally calm, steady and emotionally stable. In this work, we'll focus on the scientific aspect of meditation and the therapeutic benefits found by the scientists.

Chapter One

Types of Meditation

In this chapter, we'll have a look at the types of meditation most widely explored today by modern science. There are hundreds of types of meditation. Vijnana Bhairava, an ancient text on meditation illustrates upon one hundred and twelve types of meditation.

In the earlier ages meditation was associated with religious practices. Thanks to the Buddha, it was from his time that meditation was widely made available to public, to anyone who cared to learn and benefit from it. In recent times, especially in the west, meditation is widely practiced by people from all walks of life. If meditation could not be put under a transparent set of protocol it could not be subjected to scientific verification and its benefits would remain largely unknown.

Religious and spiritual associations are common but are not requisite for meditation practice and it should be recognized that the basis of many if not all practices is the training of the brain and body, a process that appears to have profound effects on both structure and function of human body and brain.

Meditation, as explored by the modern science can be broadly categorized under three headings:

1. Concentration based meditation or focused attention
2. Open monitoring or Mindfulness Meditation
3. Loving Kindness meditation

1. Concentration Meditation

Concentration based meditation, also called focused attention involves focusing your attention on an object such as a mantra, a mental image, certain mental construct, an abstract idea or your own breath. Trying to focus on one point often brings stress to the mind in the long term. Focused attention feels good in the beginning, but as you focus more and more you may soon become tired, because the nature of the mind is movement. Transcendental meditation falls in the category of focused attention. On concentration meditation, most researches to this day has been done on TM or transcendental meditation, which is a form of mantra meditation, involving mental repetition of a single syllable seed mantra. More than five million people have learned the technique worldwide. Since 1970, more than 600 research studies on TM have been conducted at over 250 universities and research institutions in 30 countries. Many have appeared in peer-reviewed journals. We'll come to that later.

2. Open Monitoring Meditation

Open monitoring meditation involves detached non-judgmental awareness of thoughts, feelings or sensations in your body. This type of meditation involves opening up or becoming more alert to the continuous passing stream of thoughts, images, emotions and sensations without identifying yourself with them. Such practice helps in developing non-reactive state of mind, which is the foundation for calm and peaceful state of consciousness. Here instead of narrowing the focus (concentration) practitioner becomes alert to the entire field of consciousness. Vipassana and Zen meditations belong to this category. Mindfulness meditation can fall under focused attention or open monitoring— both.

On Open Monitoring, most recent researches have been carried out on the practices of mindfulness meditation, which is widely practiced in the Buddhist traditions. Mindfulness meditation can be the most powerful kind of meditation, when you are the object of your observation. This is a variety of open-monitoring meditation. You do not need to focus in one point (here meditation is no struggle at all) but rather be aware of your thoughts, emotions, and even your physical body as a witness. Identification with your thoughts and emotions makes you forget your own self. Once you abide as the witness, the thoughts might come and go, without you identifying with them. Emotions will also come but they too will go away or dissolve into consciousness (Only natural and healthy emotions will appear eventually). Eventually concentration, better memory and happiness will be the consequence.

3. Loving Kindness Meditation

Loving-kindness is a meditation practice, which brings about positive attitudinal changes as it gradually develops the quality of 'loving-acceptance' of self and other beings. If correctly practiced, it can act as a form of self-psychotherapy, a way of healing the troubled mind to free it from its pain and confusion. Of all Buddhist meditations, loving-kindness has the immediate benefit of sweetening and changing old and deeply ingrained negative patterns of mind.

Loving-kindness meditation can be practiced by itself, or it can be practiced to support the practice of 'bare attention' to help keep the mind open and sweet. It provides the essential balance to support your mindfulness or insight meditation practice.

In fact you should combine Loving Kindness Meditation with mindfulness of breathing, or any other type of mindfulness meditation, because these practices are complementary, and that alternating these practices will prevent imbalance in your approach. Sometimes the practice of loving kindness meditation is more important than mindfulness practice — especially for people who have a tendency toward being angry or over-critical.

Loving Kindness meditation is actually a type of concentration meditation where the focus is held on the abstract idea of compassion and kindness. Loving-Kindness meditation focuses on developing feelings of goodwill, kindness and warmth towards others (Salzberg, 1997). Compassion, kindness and empathy are very basic emotions to human beings. Loving kindness meditation aims at development and culture of those basic emotions.

For the beginners, especially those who can not focus for long, and distastes sitting quietly, the Loving Kindness Meditation will be the most appropriate. It is the most natural type of meditation, because love is such an emotion that comes most naturally to all beings, human, or non human. Such a person is difficult to find who never had a person in life whom he or she could love unconditionally. It can be anyone — a loving parent, sibling, friend or spouse. It can even be a favorite pet, like a dog or a cat. And the most important thing about the Loving Kindness Meditation is that it begins from one's self. Self is the most loveable of all things and beings in this universe. In Loving Kindness Meditation, the love begins from yourself, then it expands to your loved one, and ultimately it spreads in all direction as a pure good will.

Though it sounds simple, the result of this meditation is amazing. Loving Kindness Meditation (LKM) positively impacts our emotions, our physical health, and our sense of connection with others. Not only that.

Neuroscientific meditation researcher Richard Davidson from the University of Wisconsin became interested in finding whether the positive behavioral impact of Loving Kindness positively affects our brains. He has extensively studied the effect of meditation, including LKM, on the brain. He had a simple question: Would LKM change the brain? To investigate the exact implication of this practice on the brain he invited two groups of subjects into his lab and put them under fMRI scanner to see how LKM would impact the brain. One group included those who had at least 10,000 hours of LKM in their credit and the second group included those who were interested, but new to meditation.

The results were clear. The practice of LKM changed several important brain regions: both the Insula and the temporal parietal juncture (TPJ) lit up as a result of Loving Kindness Meditation. The insula is the part of the brain responsible for our ability to empathize with others, and to make oneself aware of emotional and physical present-moment experiences. While both groups showed an increase in the insula activity, the group with 10,000 hours of experience showed significantly more activation than the other group. This group was experiencing higher levels of compassion than the non-practicing group.

Chapter Two

Meditation and Healing

Meditation in its best form is a truly holistic practice; it works on all levels of your being. Meditation has been recognized as a great healing force. It heals the body and mind, and makes us whole. When the mind is calm, alert and contented, then pure attention acts like a laser beam, which cuts through the inner debris and healing can happen at all levels.

How Meditation Heals the Body and Mind

Meditation takes us from doing to being – from thoughts and actions to silence, giving our body a very deep level of rest. The Rest is how the body heals itself. During meditation, a deep level of rest ensues, which is often deeper than what sleep can provide. During the period of deep rest, the normal metabolic functions are suspended and the body goes to recuperative and healing mode. It does the healing by throwing off the stress, fatigue, and toxins accumulated during the daily life.

The silence of pure awareness is extremely refreshing to the mind. During meditation, the mind learns to let go of the old thought-patterns, rigid habits, and stale emotional baggage of the past. When your mind is healthy, it becomes the beginning of a better physical health, because body and mind are linked.

The ancient yogis say that meditation increases Prana (the vital life energy) in the body, which is the very basis of health and well being— for both the body and the mind. When your body is alive with more Prana, you'll feel alert, energetic, and full of good humor. A lack of Prana results in lethargy, dullness and boredom.

How Meditation Increases Prana in Body and Mind

The body loves our attention, and wherever the attention flows, Prana follows. Prana follows attention or awareness like a man's shadow follows him. Meditation becomes a potent form of self-healing, when you bring your awareness to your body, which awakens every cell, filling them with fresh Prana. The more awareness you bring into your body, the stronger your immunity grows.

However, all such answers to the "How-s" come from the perspective of ancient Yogis and seers. Modern science is still far from finding the exact mechanism of how meditation acts as a healing force, apart from the experimental results of symptomatic improvement in several health criteria.

For example, a study by the University of Wisconsin's Laboratory for Affective Neuroscience reports continued changes in brain and immune functions after meditation. The scientists suggest that the stimulation of the body's immune system can account for the physical healing effects that have been reported, such as being cured of cancer or other diseases.

However, the doctors and the scientists agree on one point. That is, meditation activates the relaxation response of the body, and that has something to do with the healing it brings.

Meditation has been shown to decrease stress-related cortisol, reduce the metabolic rate, reduce respiration and heart rate, strengthen the immune system, and lead to a state of relaxation. Meditation has also been observed to increase blood flow in the brain and increase activity in the left prefrontal cortex, which is observed in happier people. This may also contribute to relaxation.

Your body is an intelligent organism; it knows how to heal itself. It is gifted by Nature with natural self-repair mechanism that fights infections repairs broken proteins, prevents aging, kills cancerous cells and maintains the homeostasis of the body. When the body gets sick, whether from the common cold or something more complicated, like heart disease, it is almost always because the body's self-repair mechanism was not working, usually because of stress.

During the time of stress, the "fight-or-flight" response is on and the self-repair mechanism is disabled. It is then when we say that the immunity of the body goes down and the body is exposed to the risk for disease. Meditation activates relaxation, when the sympathetic nervous system is turned off and the parasympathetic nervous system is turned on, and natural healing starts. We'll delve in to the details of it in the next chapters.

Chapter Three

Benefits of Meditation

The most significant health benefits of meditation are stress reduction, lower blood pressure, improved cardiovascular function, improved immunity, better sleep and the ability to stay calm and centered in the midst of all the turmoil of daily life. Subjective impacts of meditation that one can feel after a reasonably consistent practice are:

- ➢ **Greater level of relaxation**

- ➢ **Balanced state of body and mind**

- ➢ **Enhanced health and wellbeing**

- ➢ **Enhanced immunity against diseases**

- ➢ **Increased mental clarity**

- ➢ **Improved memory**

- ➢ **Increased creativity**

- ➢ **Improved capacity of decision making**

- ➢ **Reduced stress level**

> - Reduced level of anxiety

> - Increased energy level

> - Less fatigue

> - Improved sleep and relief from insomnia

> - Improved self confidence

> - Expanded level of consciousness

Meditation has the power to improve your health and immune function, increase your emotional sensitivity and emotional balance, clear and focus your mind, and strengthen your sense of spiritual connection.

General Health Benefits of Meditation

Even though meditation is a mental activity, its effects on human physiology has received much attention. The physiological effects of meditation have been documented by the scientists over the years. Before proceeding in to details, let us have a brief glance at the types of benefits documented:

Physiological Effects of Meditation

- Meditation relaxes the muscles and reduces the heart rate.

- Meditation decreases your blood pressure.

- Meditation decreases the respiratory rate.

- Meditation increases the cerebral blood flow.

- Meditation Lowers oxygen consumption.

- Meditation increases the level of your Nitric Oxide.

- Meditation increases exercise tolerance in heart patients.

- Meditation increases gray matters in the brain.

- Meditation reduces depression and enhances the immune system.

- Meditation increases brain fitness, improves memory and mental clarity.

- Meditation induces a deeper level of relaxation and reduces the stress level.

Meditation Reduces the Heart rate

Studies have indicated that heart rate slows down during quiet meditation and quickens in the moments of ecstasy during meditation (Taimni 1975). Meditations like TM, Zen, relaxation response and other calming forms of meditation generally decrease the rate of heart beat (Bono 1984; Delmonte 1984). However, very pronounced decrease in heart rate is found among long term practitioners only.

Research on the impacts of meditation on health can be classified under two broad categories: One is Preventive, which is the results that have been documented as important for disease prevention, and the other is healing aspect. Research has been carried out on different varieties of meditation to find out their impacts on the human body-mind organism. Most of the researches have been conducted in the areas of Transcendental Meditation (TM), which is a type of mantra meditation involving focused attention, Mindfulness Meditation and Loving Kindness Meditation.

Meditation Improves Memory & Brain Fitness

Studies had demonstrated that regular meditators do have consistent, notable structural differences in their brains, specifically a thickening of the cerebral cortex in areas associated with attention and emotional integration.

Participating in an eight-week mindfulness meditation program appears to make measurable changes in brain regions associated with memory, sense of self, empathy, and stress. In a study, a team led by Harvard-affiliated researchers at Massachusetts General Hospital (MGH) reported that meditation produced changes over time in the brain's gray matter. The research lead by Sara W. Lazar and team found that practicing mindfulness meditation actually lead to increases in regional brain gray matter density in different brain areas.

The study senior author Sara Lazar of the MGH Psychiatric Neuroimaging Research Program and   a Harvard   Medical School instructor in psychology says,

"Although the practice of meditation is associated with a sense of peacefulness and physical relaxation, practitioners have long claimed that meditation also provides cognitive and psychological benefits that persist throughout the day. This study demonstrates that changes in brain structure may underlie some of these reported improvements and that people are not just feeling better because they are spending time relaxing."

For their study, magnetic resonance (MR) images were taken of the brain structure of 16 study participants two weeks before and after they took part in the eight-week Mindfulness-Based Stress Reduction (MBSR) Program at the University of Massachusetts Center for Mindfulness. The program included weekly meetings that included practice of

33

mindfulness meditation — which focuses on nonjudgmental awareness of sensations, feelings, and state of mind, and the participants received audio recordings for guided meditation practice.

Meditation group participants reported spending an average of 27 minutes each day practicing mindfulness exercises. The analysis of MR images, which focused on areas where meditation-associated differences were seen in earlier studies, found increased gray-matter density in the hippocampus, known to be important for learning and memory, and in structures associated with self-awareness, compassion, and introspection.

Meditation in Pain Management

Rapid breathing is controlled by the sympathetic nervous system. It's part of the "fight or flight" response — the part activated by stress. In contrast, slow, deep breathing actually stimulates the opposing parasympathetic reaction — the one that calms us down. Meditation, any type of meditation makes the breathing slower and deeper automatically. It creates an effect of natural, spontaneous pranayama that relaxes us. Slow deep breathing (approximately 6 breaths per minute) has analgesic effects.

Recent research performed by a scientist at Barrow Neurological Institute at St. Joseph's Hospital and Medical Center has shown that controlled breathing at a slowed rate can significantly reduce feelings of pain.

The research was led by Arthur (Bud) Craig, PhD, at Barrow, and was done in collaboration with investigators in the Department of Psychology at Arizona State University. It was published in the journal PAIN (Zautra et al. 2010), the refereed journal of the International Association for the Study of Pain (IASP). The findings offer an explanation for prior reports that mindful Zen meditation has beneficial effects on pain.

Meditation Improves Immunity

There is increasing evidence that meditative practice also favorably affects the immune system. Meditation actually increases the immunity of the body against diseases. Slow, deep breathing practiced in yogic meditation can influence the autonomic nervous system. A better understanding of meditation's effects on the autonomic nervous system and the immune system and their dynamic links to the central nervous system will help us understand better how meditation increases the immunity.

How Meditation Increases Immunity?

Psychological states such as stress affect the functioning of the immune system. The immune system is indirectly under the influence of the central nervous system via hormonal signaling and through activity of the autonomic nervous system.

Meditation stimulates the parasympathetic nervous system which creates deep relaxation response to body and the mind. A comprehensive study conducted by the researchers of the Harvard Medical School under the leadership of Dr. Herbert Benson (Benson, Beary, and Carol 1974) shows that deep relaxation changes our bodies on a

36

genetic level. What the researchers at Harvard Medical School discovered is that in long term practitioners of deeper relaxation techniques such as meditation, far more 'disease-fighting genes' were active, compared to those who do not practice. In particular, they found genes were switched on that protect from disorders such as pain, infertility, high blood pressure and even rheumatoid arthritis. The changes, the researchers say, were induced by the relaxation effect, a phenomenon that could be just as powerful as any medical drug, but without any side effects.

This experiment shows just how responsive the genes are to our behavior, mood and environment, and they can switch on just as easily as they can switch off. The Harvard researchers asked the control group to start practicing meditation inducing relaxation every day. After two months, their bodies began to change. The genes that help fight inflammation, kill diseased cells and protect the bodies from auto-immune diseases began to switch on.

More encouraging still, the benefits of relaxation effect were found to increase with regular practice. This research is pivotal in proving how a person's state of mind affects the body on a physical and genetic level.

Davidson et al. (2003) found faster peak rise for the antibody response to a flu shot among healthy meditators who underwent an 8-week mindfulness-based stress reduction (MBSR) training course in open monitoring meditation than among non-meditators. Increased number and increased activity of lymphocyte T and other natural killer cells (NK cells) have also been found in HIV patients after MBSR training. In a recent study, (Pace et al. 2009) assessed the effect of compassion meditation (in which one works at developing altruistic emotions and behaviors towards all living beings) on the immune response and found a negative correlation between the amount of meditation practice and induced stress immune response.

Davidson et al. (2003) also found that left-sided anterior oscillatory activity of the brain is positively correlated with activity of the immune system after meditation practice, assessing through the quantity of natural killer (NK) cells.

Meditative practices have been linked to a number of aspects of immune functioning in healthy adults, including immune cell stability, inflammation in response to stress, and responsiveness to a vaccine. Adults with previous meditation experience were recruited for a 3-month-long study on the effects of combined open monitoring and kindness-and-compassion meditation training on telomerase activity in immune cells. Telomerase is an enzyme that maintains the protective "end caps" on DNA that promote genomic stability and prevent mutation; higher levels of telomerase are linked to lower levels of stress and better health (Epel, 2009) (Epel et al. 2009). Meditators showed greater immune cell telomerase activity at the end of the study relative to age, sex and BMI-matched control participants (Jacobs et al. 2011).

Other evidence also links open monitoring and loving-kindness to immune functioning. Healthy college students were randomly assigned to 10 weeks of either loving-kindness training or, as an active control, a health education discussion group. At the end of the study, all participants completed the Trier Social Stress Test and blood plasma samples were taken to measure changes in interleukin-6 (IL-6), a marker of inflammation, in response to the stressor. The two groups did not differ in IL-6 responses; however, within the meditation group, more time spent meditating predicted lower levels of IL-6 in response to the stressor (Pace et al. 2009).

In a more direct measure of immune functioning, 8 weeks of mindfulness-based stress reduction (MBSR) training, which involves open monitoring and focused attention practices, predicted a greater rise in antibody titers in response to the influenza vaccine for adult meditators relative to participants in a wait-list control group (Davidson et al., 2003).

Chapter Four

Meditation and Happiness Factor

Neuroscientists say happiness is the result of brain activity. We have already discussed how meditation makes us feel happier by deactivating the "Me" center of the brain and reducing mind wandering.

Human happiness and ability to enjoy life is very much dependent on the function of our pre-frontal cortex (PFC). The 'happy' center of our brain is in our left hemisphere. Happiness is associated with a greater activity in the left prefrontal region, while negative emotions are linked to a greater activity in the right prefrontal cortex.

The more activation in the left prefrontal cortex is associated with more positive emotions and happiness. Meditation increases blood flow in the PFC. A greater activation of the left prefrontal brain compared to the right part of the brain happens during meditation, and more so, when the meditation is focused on loving-kindness and compassion.

The feeling of happiness and wellbeing has also something to do with the chemicals called neurotransmitters. Meditation practices act on the hypothalamic–pituitary–adrenal axis (HPA) axis to reduce cortisol levels in plasma as well as reduce sympathetic nervous system tone, increase vagal activity, and elevate brain GABA levels. People with GABA dominant brains are often good organizers. They can handle complex and stressful occupations. The neurotransmitters GABA and serotonin enable the brain to control anxious thoughts. Meditation also decreases Cortisol and Norepinephrine, which are related to stress.

What happens in the brain during meditation?

In this context, it must be noted that happiness isn't simply a pleasurable feeling. It's much more complex than that. Research has also implicated other hormones, like progesterone, oxytocin and testosterone, in producing other aspects of happiness, like a sense of well-being and connectedness with others.

The emotional effects of sitting quieting and going within are profound. The deep state of rest produced by meditation triggers the brain to release neurotransmitters, including dopamine, serotonin, oxytocin, and endorphins. Each of these naturally occurring brain chemicals has been linked to different aspects of happiness:

Neurologists know that Dopamine plays a key role in the brain's ability to experience pleasure, feel rewarded, and maintain focus.

Serotonin has a calming effect. It eases tension and helps us feel less stressed and more relaxed and focused. Low levels of this ncurotransmitter have been linked to migraines, anxiety, bipolar disorder, apathy, feelings of worthlessness, fatigue, and insomnia.

Oxytocin (the same chemical whose levels rise during sexual arousal and breastfeeding), is a pleasure hormone. It creates feelings of calm, contentment, and security, while reducing fear and anxiety.

Endorphins are the chemicals that create the exhilaration commonly labelled as "the runner's high." These neurotransmitters play many roles related to wellbeing, including decreasing feelings of pain and reducing the side effects of stress.

Meditation Increases GABA, Melatonin, and Serotonin.

Meditation activates the brain to release neurotransmitters, including dopamine, serotonin, oxytocin, and endorphins. Each of these naturally occurring brain chemicals has been linked to different aspects of happiness.

Chapter Five

Meditation and Gray Matter in the Brain

Gray matter (or grey matter) in the brain is directly responsible for memory, seeing, hearing, executive functions, impulse control, emotions and speech. As age increase gray matter in the brain decreases. However, meditation, yoga, omega-3 and many other things can increase the gray matters in the brain (Wilson 2015). In this section we focus on the techniques and methods to increase the gray matters in the brain.

What are Gray Matters?

The central nervous system is made up of two kinds of tissue: gray matter and white matter. Gray matters are the darker tissue of the brain and spinal cord, consisting mainly of nerve cell bodies and branching dendrites. Gray matters look like ash-gray under a microscope. These are composed of neuron's cell bodies and synapses, as well as the supporting network of glia that help keep neurons alive. The color difference between gray matter and white matter arises mainly from the whiteness of myelin. In living brain, gray matter actually has a gray-brown color which comes from capillary blood vessels and neuronal cell bodies. Ratio of the volume of gray-matter to white-matter in the cerebral hemispheres (20 yrs. old) is about 1.3.

Location of the Gray Matters

Gray matter mainly located on the surface of the cerebral cortex, and on surface of the cerebellum. It is also found in the deeper parts of the cerebrum, and hippocampus. Grey matter is present in the brain as well as in the spinal cord. It travels down the spinal cord in three gray columns.

Functions and Characteristic of Gray Matters

The gray matter includes regions of the brain involved in muscle control, and sensory perception such as seeing and hearing, memory, emotions, speech, decision making, and self-control. While 20% of all oxygen taken in by the body goes to the brain, 95% of that goes specifically into the grey matter. Scientists observed significant positive correlations between gray matter volume in elderly persons and measures of semantic and short-term memory.

The more gray matter you have in the decision-making, thought-processing part of your brain, the better your ability to evaluate rewards and consequences. Normally, gray matter represents information processing centers in the brain, and white matter represents the networking of – or connections between – these processing centers.

The larger the animal, the more convoluted this grey matter is. Small animals such as the marmoset tend to have smooth brains, while in larger mammals such as the whale or elephant the grey matter is highly convoluted.

How Gray Matters is Related to Age

Age is negatively associated with gray matter volume. Elderly people show lower volumes of gray matters in the brain. Gray matters are directly linked to memory and reduction of gray matters causes memory problems for elderly people. Aging is associated with cognitive decline, diminished brain function. Brain function depends on large-scale distributed networks, and aging disrupted the structural and functional brain connectivity. However, scientists observed that with proper yoga, meditation, exercises and diet can increase the gray matter in the brain.

Reasons for Decreasing Gray-Matter in the Brain

Some of the most common reasons for reducing gray matters are as follows:

1. Gray matter declines steadily as we grow older from the age of adolescence. Studies have identified areas such as the insula as being especially vulnerable to age-related losses in gray matter of older adults.

2. Media multitasking reduces the number of gray matters. Media multitasking means simultaneous use of media. Media multitasking involves using TV, the Web, radio, mobile, telephone, print, or any other

media in conjunction with another. Loh KK (Loh and Kanai 2014) observed heavier media-multitasking worsen the cognitive control tasks and individuals with higher Media Multitasking Index (MMI) scores had smaller gray matter density in the anterior cingulate cortex (ACC).

3. Smokers lose grey-matter and cognitive function at a greater rate than non-smokers. Chronic smokers who quit during the study lost fewer brain cells and retained better intellectual function than those who continued to smoke. Regular use of the drug seems to shrink the brain's gray matter.

4. Stress in early life is associated with increased rates of mood and anxiety disorders in adulthood. Exposed to childhood maltreatment, reduces gray matter volume within the hippocampus and other areas.

5. Chronic stress reduces gray matter volume in the pre-frontal area.

How Meditation Helps to Increase Gray Matter

Mindfulness Meditation is the simple way to increases gray matter volume in the brain. Mindfulness meditation is basically paying precise, nonjudgmental attention to the details of our moment to moment experience. Mindfulness meditation is often practiced sitting with eyes closed, cross-legged on a cushion, or on a chair, with the back straight. You can put your attention on the breath as it goes in and out the nostrils. Or it may be practiced by observing the movement of the abdomen when breathing in and out. As new thoughts come up, you can return to focusing on the object of meditation, such as the breathing. You can passively in a non-judgmental way notice the mind as it wandered. This type of meditation can be done for the periods of 10 to 15 minutes or so a day.

The hippocampus, or more precisely the left hippocampus is primarily responsible for its role in memory, contribute to our usual mind-wandering. It is also important to note that stress hurts the hippocampus. Nonjudgmental awareness of mindfulness meditation reduces mind-wandering as well as stress allowing the recovery of the hippocampal neurons.

Chapter Six

Meditation and White Matter in the Brain

White matter is that element of the brain made of cells called 'axons' that connect one to the other so that nerves can communicate. White matters are the subway of the brain – connecting different regions of grey matter in the cerebrum to one another. The white matter mostly remains deeper underneath the surface. Without functioning white matter, the brain could be like a group of people in closeness to each other but unable to communicate with each other. In contrast to gray matter, in which the cell bodies of neurons dominate, the term white matter refers to areas of the brain where there is a predominance of axons coated with myelin. White matter occupies almost half of the human brain.

Traditionally white matter has been thought not to change after the period in development when axonal migration and myelination have taken place. However, this concept has been changing. Studies in aged humans show that myelin begins to degrade in aging and that learning new skills improves the integrity of white matter in the brain by slowing loss of myelin (Engvig et al. 2011). Studies have shown that two hours of game training can change in white matter structure in the human brain (Hofstetter et al. 2013).

As little as 2–4 weeks of meditation training can change the white matter in the brain (Posner, Tang, and Lynch 2014). Meditation influences frontal brain rhythms, and the consequence of these rhythms on protease secretion that influence glial cells in forming the basis of white matter change.

Chapter Seven

Researches in Different Types of Meditation

As there are different types of meditation, to scientifically assess the effect of meditation on the health and wellbeing of a practitioner, the researchers needed to conduct research on specific type of meditation and find its effect on the practitioner. While almost all kinds of meditation can be beneficial, it's important to note that different types of meditation practices engage the mind in different ways and produce very different results, and scientific research showing specific benefits from one type of practice does not apply to all other practices. For example, Transcendental Meditation is the only practice recommended by the American Heart Association for the reduction of high blood pressure, based on the AHA's own research into different forms of meditation (mindfulness was not found to have a significant effect on hypertension). TM is also the only meditation found in clinical trials to reduce heart attack and stroke. "Mindfulness" (or "open monitoring") is one specific process of meditation, with its own EEG brainwave pattern (theta), that have been proven useful to cure depression. Loving Kindness meditation has been proven effective in chronic pain, migraine and schizophrenia. A considerable number of researches have been carried out on various specific types of meditation practices, such as TM, Mindfulness, or Loving Kindness meditation.

Research in TM

The first ground-breaking research in meditation took place in 60s decade. The year 1968 marked as a real turning point for scientific research in to meditation, when a group of Transcendental meditation practitioners turned up at the Harvard Medical School, and they offered themselves to be studied. They claimed that they could reduce their blood pressure with the practice.

Fortunately for them, and for the benefits of generations to come, Herbert Benson, then a cardiologist at Harvard, agreed to a study. Dr. Benson was so impressed with what he found in his study that he published a book on it. "The Relaxation Response" was published in 1975 by Dr. Benson and Miriam Klipper, which by 1986 became a best-seller that the clinical psychologists started recommending to their patients.

Transcendental meditation (TM) is the first meditation practice that came out with comprehensive scientific evidence of wide-ranging beneficial effects. Initially, TM has demonstrated to reduce tension and increase intelligence and performance and that long-term practice reverses the aging process. Subsequently it was shown to be preventive as well as curative in a wide variety of illnesses: CNS, CVS, Endocrine, Respiratory, Metabolic, Immune system and Inter body system and found to be effective in hypertension and wide variety of cardiovascular diseases.

Dr. Herbert Benson conducted a series of clinical tests on meditators from various disciplines, including Transcendental Meditation and Tibetan Buddhism, Benson is a pioneer in mind/body medicine, one of the first Western physicians to bring spirituality and healing into medicine. Since then, meditation has become a major focus of research for experts in multiple disciplines in major US and European universities. Leading Universities in the USA and Europe have established dedicated research centers in to meditation.

Benefits of TM on Cardiovascular Health

Many randomized controlled trials (RCTs) have shown following results:

1. In a nine-year RCT of patients with coronary heart disease, TM led to a 48% reduction in the rate of major clinical events (all-cause mortality plus non-fatal myocardial infarction and stroke) compared to controls who received education on risk factor reduction, including diet modification and exercise.

2. TM was more effective in reducing mild hypertension than progressive muscular relaxation or a 'usual care' programme.

3. TM reduced blood pressure effectively in both sexes and across a range of risk subgroups; cost-effectiveness compared favourably with drugs.

4. Follow-up studies confirmed sustained blood pressure reductions with TM.

5. TM reduced carotid artery atherosclerosis compared to controls who received health education.

6. Pooled data from two randomized studies on hypertensive older people showed that TM was associated with a 23% reduction in all-cause mortality and a 30% decrease in cardiovascular deaths.

7. In patients with stable coronary heart disease, TM decreased both blood pressure and insulin resistance - key components of the 'metabolic syndrome' associated with many major disorders of modern society, including CHD (coronary heart disease), type 2 diabetes, and hypertensive disease. TM also increased stability of the cardiac autonomic nervous system

8. TM improved functional capacity and quality of life in patients with chronic heart failure. TM subjects also showed reduced depression and had fewer hospitalizations.

9. In university students, TM reduced blood pressure, and also decreased total psychological distress, anxiety, depression, and anger/hostility; and improved coping.

10. In pre-hypertensive adolescents, TM improved blood pressure at rest, during acute laboratory stress, and during normal daily activity.

11. TM decreased left ventricular mass in pre-hypertensive adolescents compared to a control group receiving health education, indicating reduction of an early sign of left ventricular hypertrophy, (the strongest predictor of cardiovascular mortality apart from age).

Controlled research on TM has also found: improved exercise tolerance in angina patients with documented coronary lesions;

reduction of elevated cholesterol; improvements in clinical and ECG variables in patients with cardiac syndrome; lower cortisol levels and reduced cardiovascular risk factors in post-menopausal women.

Research in Mindfulness Meditation

Mindfulness meditation - another important type of Buddhist meditation- has been a subject of focus and widely studied in the recent times by the scientists. Open monitoring or mindfulness meditation has been practiced for more than 2500 years or so in the Asian countries since the time of the Buddha, who is known to make the teaching popular among his disciples. But it is only in the last 20 years or so, that the beneficial effects of mindfulness meditation techniques in relieving physical pain symptoms and mental distress have been subjected to modern scientific scrutiny.

In a study conducted at five middle schools in Belgium, involving about 400 students (13 ~ 20 years old), Professor Filip Raes concludes: "students who follow an in-class mindfulness program report reduced indications of depression, anxiety and stress up to six months later. Moreover, these students were less likely to develop pronounced depression-like symptoms."

Another study, from the University of California, made with patients with past depression, published in the JAMA network concluded that mindfulness meditation decreases ruminative thinking and dysfunctional beliefs among patients.

Mindfulness Meditation for Mental Health

Mindfulness meditation has specially been noticed to improve mental health and brain fitness. In the year 2008 Oxford mindfulness center was founded within Oxford University's department of psychiatry under the guidance of professor Mark Williams, one of the pioneers in mindfulness based cognitive therapy. It has been at the forefront of research and development in the field of mindfulness in UK. Now they use mindfulness meditation as a therapy, termed as mindfulness based cognitive therapy (MBCT). MBCT has become a treatment of choice for the prevention of recurrent depression in the UK National health service. The effectiveness of mindfulness meditation has been clinically proven to reduce suicidality in depression and emotional turbulence in bipolar disorder.

Researchers in the oxford university have found that: In patients with three or more previous episodes of depression, MBCT reduces the recurrence rate over 12 months by 40 to 50 percent compared to usual care. MBCT has been proved as effective as antidepressants for reducing recurrence.

How does this happen? According to the cognitive research, those who have suffered from depression already are particularly vulnerable to mood-related triggers that send them in to an auto-pilot mode, inducing cycles of repetitive negative thinking and thereby causing relapse. With MBCT, the patients develop the ability to recognize and disengage from negative thought patterns and forge a new relationship to themselves and their surroundings.

MBCT uses those elements of CBT (Cognitive Behavioral Therapy), along with mindfulness, that decentralize thoughts. They train their patients to learn that "Thoughts are not facts," and "I am not my thoughts". Unlike CBT, the emphasis is not changing the content of the thoughts; instead using the mindfulness meditation they train their subjects to focus on changing the awareness of and the relation to their thoughts. As a result the participants discover what makes them vulnerable to downward mood spirals, explore ways of releasing themselves from the auto-pilot, and discover a new way to relate to themselves and the world, noticing the present moment rather than living in the past or worrying about the future.

The benefits of mindfulness in preventing serious depression and emotional disorder have also been proven by numerous clinical trials in the USA.

Mindfulness Meditation for Stress Reduction

Dr. John Kabat-Zinn applied mindfulness-based practices to put distance between the patient and his cognitive, emotional, and sensory experiences Kabat-Zinn's mindfulness-based stress reduction (MBSR) program has become widely popular since about 1970 (Kabat-Zinn J. 1990) and is now often accepted in clinical settings.

Almost all the varieties of meditation succeed in reducing stress level in the body and mind. Over 200 medical institutions around the world introduced Mindfulness Based Stress Reduction Program.

Chapter Eight

Meditation and Cardiovascular Health

The impact of meditation on cardiovascular health was highlighted in the interesting article published in the International journal of Cardiology on July issue in 2013. The research paper by Dr. Stephen Olex, Dr. Andrew Newberg and Vincent Figueredo was titled "Meditation Should a Cardiologist care?" (Olex, Newberg, and Figueredo 2013). The purport of this question is obvious. As a human being, you may be interested in meditation, because anybody meditating for a reasonable time will attest to the fact that meditation provides a sense of general wellbeing, and if you believe in a higher power or God, meditation is a way to connect to that supreme cosmic intelligence. But, as a cardiologist, should you care for meditation? Or, will you prescribe it to your patients? That is the question asked by the authors of the research paper, and they provided the answer. They concluded that available evidence suggests that meditation may exert beneficial effects on autonomic tone, autonomic reflexes, and it actually decreases blood pressure acutely and after long term practice. In addition, meditation has the potential to positively influence the cardiovascular system through the mind-heart connection and the anti-inflammatory reflex. There is limited but promising data to suggest that meditation based interventions can have beneficial effects on patients with established cardiovascular disease.

Long back in 1984, Delmonte (Delmonte 1984) had concluded that meditation as an intervention strategy was successful with anxiety and hypertension.

Meditative interventions have been found to be beneficial in treating various clinical conditions. These include- hypertension cardiovascular disorders; pain syndromes and musculoskeletal diseases; respiratory disorders and immunological disorders.

Between 1970 and 1990s an extensive research initiative led by Orme-Jhonson (Orme-Johnson et al. 2006) produced a vast databank of 508 studies reporting on the evidence supporting a possible hypo-metabolic fourth state of consciousness beyond the usual waking, dream and deep sleep states. It also documented a reduction in medical conditions such as asthma, angina and high blood pressure.

A number of different meditative practices have been linked to positive cardiovascular outcomes. Three months of MBSR training for healthy led to significantly greater decreases in blood pressure relative to both life-skills training and health education control conditions. In a meta-analysis of the effects of meditation on adults diagnosed with hypertension, transcendental meditation, a form of focused attention involving chanting a personalized mantra, was more effective than progressive muscle relaxation in producing a clinically significant reduction in blood pressure.

However, most remarkable research on the effect of meditation on heart health involves studies on transcendental meditation. In recent years, a multicentre American team has been provided grants totaling over $25 million, principally from the US National Institutes of Health, for research on TM and cardiovascular health in older African-Americans (a high-risk group for vascular disease).

An interesting study was carried out under the leadership of Dr. Robert Schneider in 2012 which was published in the Journal of American Heart Association(Schneider et al. 2012). The study was labeled as: Stress reduction in the secondary prevention of cardiovascular disease: randomized, controlled trial of transcendental meditation and health education in Blacks. In America the African-American populations or the Blacks have disproportionately high rates of cardiovascular disease. Psychosocial stress may contribute to this disparity.

Psychosocial stress is associated with the onset and progression of cardiovascular disease in the general population. Stress reduction with the Transcendental Meditation program has been shown to beneficially affect cardiovascular risk factors, e.g., hypertension, psychological stress, substance abuse, insulin resistance, myocardial ischemia, left ventricular mass and carotid atherosclerosis.

This study under guidance of Dr. Schneider was a randomized, controlled trial of 201 black men and women with coronary heart disease who were randomized to the TM program or health education. The primary end point was the composite of all-cause mortality, myocardial infarction, or stroke. Secondary end points included the composite of cardiovascular mortality, revascularizations, and cardiovascular hospitalizations; blood pressure; psychosocial stress factors; and lifestyle behaviors.

During an average follow-up of 5.4 years, there was a 48% risk reduction in the primary end point in the TM group. The TM group also showed a 24% risk reduction in the secondary end point. There were reductions in systolic blood pressure and anger expression. They concluded that adding stress-reducing Transcendental Meditation to usual care in patients with coronary heart disease resulted in a 48% reduction in the risk for cardiovascular clinical events, that is, mortality, myocardial infarction, and stroke during >5 years of follow-up.

TM was applied by another study was conducted in 2009 by Dr. Schneidar, Dr. Merz and the team(Tanner et al. 2009). The result was published in the journal of American heart association. The studies indicate that this meditation technique reduces risk factors and can slow or reverse the progression of what they call pathophysiological changes underlying cardiovascular disease. Studies with this technique have revealed reductions in blood pressure and surrogate markers of disease–carotid artery intima-media thickness, left ventricular hypertrophy and stress-induced myocardial ischemia.

"What this is saying is that mind-body interventions can have an effect as big as conventional medications, such as statins," says Dr. Schneider.

Now there is a consensus among the doctors and researchers that lifestyle plays a crucial role in preventing a heart attack or recovering from one. But how does meditation help the patients of coronary heart disease or lower the risk of myocardial infarction in the patients of coronary heart disease? Myocardial infarction occurs when an artery leading to the heart becomes completely blocked and the heart doesn't get enough blood or oxygen, causing cells in that area of the heart to die. It is mostly caused by blood clots, which are in turn caused by atherosclerosis (stiffening and narrowing of the arteries). High blood fats (triglycerides) and LDL or "bad" cholesterol form plaque inside the arteries, narrowing the passageway and reducing the amount of blood that can flow through. Does meditation acts as beta blockers that dilate the arteries? Possibly so.

Cardiologist Dr. Dean Ornish in the clinical trial published in 1990 in the journal Lancet has demonstrated that some of his patients experienced a dissolving (regression) of atherosclerotic plaques that had been obstructing blood flows through their coronary arteries. Dr. Ornish has shown that a lifestyle modification program of regular meditation, a vegetarian diet and exercises can very successfully stop building up of cholesterol and plaques in coronary arteries.

"It appears that Transcendental Meditation is a technique that turns on the body's own pharmacy – to repair and maintain itself." said lead researcher Dr Robert Schneider, director of the Institute for Natural Medicine and Prevention in Iowa. Dr Schneider added: "Transcendental Meditation may reduce heart disease risks for both healthy people and those with diagnosed heart conditions."

The reason for the overall health benefits of meditation are attributed to a factor termed as the Relaxation Response. The causes of meditation's therapeutic effects are a part of general relaxation produced by parasympathetic dominance. Conditions responsible for the relaxation response in any meditation technique are: a quiet environment, a passive attitude, decreased muscle tones and use of mental devices to facilitate shift away from the ordinary random thought process. Taylor et al. suggested that nonetheless there are findings that meditation reduces stress as indicated in lower level of adrenal hormones and lactates.

Major benefit of meditation related to coronary heart disease comes from meditator's increased capability to cope with stress. **What is stress?**

Stress is not the event, but the residual physiological imbalance, or impression left in the nervous system, (known for millennia in the Yoga tradition as samskara – or scars) which then inhibits our quality of performance in every aspect of life.

Though we tend to define some events as stressful, psychologists have found that since different people interpret the same event differently, it is not the events themselves, but our interpretation of the events as challenging, terrible and stressful— we all know all types of labeling that mind does — is responsible for the effect that the event does on our bodies – creates the fight or flight response – which is known as stress. Most types of meditation give us a certain detachment to look at an event objectively without getting too much involved in the interpretation of the event.

Stress hormones including cortisol and adrenaline are responsible for temporarily changing the functioning of the whole body. Stored glucose and fats are released for energy, heart rate increases, blood pressure rises, muscles tense, and oxygen consumption increases, whilst other processes not needed at that time are suppressed, such as digestion, cellular repair and sexual functioning. Effects in the brain cause heightened emotional responses and reduced decision making processes. Research suggests that prolonged stress contributes to high blood pressure, promotes the formation of artery-clogging deposits precipitating myocardial infarction.

Meditation Reduces the Risk Factor of Coronary Heart Disease

An interesting study was carried out by Dr. C. Noel Bairey Merz, MD and his team at the Division of Cardiology, Department of Medicine, Cedars-Sinai Research Institute, of Los Angeles, CA that verified the viability of meditation as an important intervention method in CHD(Paul-Labrador et al. 2006).

The metabolic syndrome, characterized by the clustering of hypertension, dyslipidemia, visceral obesity, and insulin resistance, is now regarded as a risk factor for cardiovascular morbidity and mortality and is recognized as a new means of detecting coronary heart disease (CHD) risk. Insulin resistance is regarded by many researchers as a key component of the metabolic syndrome, which is related to visceral obesity and hypertension. Because metabolic syndrome is thought to be a contributor to coronary heart disease (CHD), the components of the syndrome have been identified as possible therapeutic targets. Previous data implicate neurohumoral activation related to psychosocial stress as a contributor to the metabolic syndrome.

Randomized controlled trials of transcendental meditation (TM) have demonstrated a blood pressure–lowering effect similar to a first-line antihypertensive medication compared with a control intervention of health education (HE).

Patients were recruited from a supervised cardiac exercise and rehabilitation program at Cedars-Sinai Medical Center and the surrounding community. They included women and men older than 18 years, with CHD documented by prior myocardial infarction, coronary artery bypass surgery, coronary angiography, or angioplasty. Exclusion criteria consisted of unstable coronary syndromes and acute myocardial infarction in the preceding 3 months. The aim of this study published in the JAMA in 2006 was to evaluate the efficacy of transcendental meditation (TM) on components of the metabolic syndrome and CHD.

They conducted a randomized, placebo-controlled clinical trial of 16 weeks of TM or active control treatment (health education), matched for frequency and time, at an academic medical center in a total of 103 subjects with stable CHD. Main outcome measures included blood pressure, lipoprotein profile, and insulin resistance determined by homeostasis model assessment. The TM group had beneficial changes in adjusted systolic blood pressure, insulin resistance, and heart rate variability compared with the health education group.

This led them to conclude that the use of TM for 16 weeks in CHD patients improved blood pressure and insulin resistance components of the metabolic syndrome as well as cardiac autonomic nervous system tone compared with a control group receiving health education. These results suggest that TM may modulate the physiological response to stress and improve CHD risk factors, which may be a novel therapeutic target for the treatment of CHD.

Meditation Reduced Atherosclerosis

This was published in American Journal of Cardiology, April 2002 issue. The study's subjects with multiple risk factors for cardiovascular disease were found to have substantially reduced atherosclerosis through a multi-modality treatment program derived from a system of traditional medicine that included daily Transcendental Meditation practice.

Another randomized, controlled clinical trial showed that the daily practice of the Transcendental Meditation technique was associated with or decreased narrowing of the arteries in the heart and brain in high-risk hypertensive adults, thereby decreasing the risk of heart attack and stroke.

An eight months study of 21 patients with coronary artery disease by J. W. Zamarra and associates, published in American Journal of Cardiology, found that the patients taught TM had a 14.7% improvement in treadmill stress test performance compared to the control group.

Meditation for the Management of Myocardial Infarction Patients

If a person survives myocardial infarction, the medical term for heart attack, it can cause him a serious heart muscle weakness called cardiomyopathy. Due to cardiomyopathy, a person can experience terrible shortness of breath caused by their lungs filling up with fluid a condition known as congestive heart failure. In 2007 Ravi Jayadevappa and fellow researchers at the university of Pennsylvania reported a randomized control trial of 23 African Americans with congestive heart failure, who were randomized to either a TM or a health education group. This six months long study found that TM resulted in improved exercise capacity and feelings of well being in the patients with congestive heart failure. Also, the TM group had fewer hospitalizations during the study period.

An interesting study was published in the Journal of Cardiovascular nursing that stressed upon the Influence of Psychosocial Factors and Biopsychosocial Interventions on Outcomes after Myocardial Infarction. It says that the patients of myocardial infarction often suffers from psychosocial factors such as depression, coronary-prone behavior, hostility, anxiety, anger, and stress that aggravates the risk of cardiac death and illness. They suggested meditation and relaxation exercises as preventive care.

Actually patients and doctors often bear testimony to the fact that the patients that undergo angioplasty or bypass surgery are often victims of depression and anxiety.

Meditation can serve them as a grounding factor helping them to live in the present moment and thus contributes to a feeling of well being.

Chapter Nine

Meditation and Stress Reduction

Meditating every day can make a huge difference in how you approach life situations, how you interact with your spouse, relations, friends and colleagues, and how personally you take things. Meditation is long known to enrich your life by enhancing compassion, allowing you to see things differently with more clarity, having a clear assessment of yourself and connecting you with the center of calm within you. Meditation enriches your life by reducing anxiety, making you more centered and empathetic.

Stress has been a constant companion of the fast paced modern lifestyle, which makes people susceptible to various illnesses by weakening their immune system, you know. Meditation is gaining in popularity as a means of treating stress and enhancing psychological wellbeing. We all know that of various descriptions is regarded as a probable etiological factor in common health problems including heart disease, anxiety disorder, and chronic depression. A study done in 1998 by the Journal of Occupational and Environmental Medicine found that 50-58%of all illness are stress related. In order to cope with stress more efficiently we need to develop a greater sense of self-awareness. The key to achieving this self awareness lies in shifting one's attention from the immediate external environment to one's internal environment. Meditation, any type of meditation, does just that.

Recent studies indicate that mindfulness meditation training interventions reduce stress and improve stress-related health outcomes. Studies show that a 3-day intensive mindfulness meditation training intervention (relative to a well-matched 3-day relaxation training intervention without a mindfulness component) reduced right amygdale activity in a sample of stressed unemployed community adults (n = 35). Generally, stress may increase amygdale activity brief training in mindfulness meditation could reverse these effects (Taren et al. 2015).

Before going in to details of how meditation helps the functioning of the different organs of the body and how it improves different health conditions, it is important to recognize that most illness have a psychosomatic component. A growing body of research is acknowledging this in recent times. Any illness can be called psychosomatic condition when dysfunction or structural damage in bodily organs occurs through inappropriate activation of the autonomic nervous system and the endocrine glands.

You might be acquainted with the name of the neuroscientist Dr. Candice Pert, who wrote the book "The Molecules of Emotion"(Pert 2004). Dr. Candice Pert's research has established a biochemical basis for self awareness and consciousness, linking mind and body as one. The studies have demonstrated that our emotions are formulated in the cells of the body and the brain through chemicals binding to specific receptors at the surface of the cells. Thus they transmit information in to the cells. The changes in the cells are then transmitted by nerve impulses across the cell membrane to produce corresponding change in your mood, behavior and physical activity. Through this mechanism repressed emotions are stored. (Pert, 1997, Butlin, 2001)(Pert 2004).

Dr. Candice Pert's research threw new light on how stress and negative emotions adversely affects the subjects. Dr. Pert's research can throw light on how a mental activity such as meditation can cure several illnesses that are by-products of stress.

How Meditation Reduces Anxiety?

The more you meditate, the less anxious you become. How? To understand this, you need to know about the "Me" Center (technically, it is the medial prefrontal cortex) of your brain. This is the part of brain that gives us identity and it processes information relating to ourselves and our experiences.

The medial prefrontal cortex area becomes active when you are daydreaming, thinking about the future, engaging in social interactions, reflecting on yourself, inferring other people's state of mind or feeling empathy for others.

This "Me" center often engages in creating emotional assumptions and false stories in the way of processing an information. For the non-meditators, this section of the brain, called the "Me" Center, remains very actively and strongly connected to the neural pathways from the Insula, the part of the brain that monitors bodily sensations and is involved in experiencing "gut-level" feelings. The neural connection between the "Me" center and the Amygdala, the "fear center" of the brain is also very strong for the non-meditators. So, when they experience a scary or upsetting sensation, it triggers a strong reaction in their "Me" Center, which readily create an assumption of danger (which is often wrong), making them feel scared and under attack. As a result stress response takes place and various stress hormones are secreted, making you anxious and stressed.

When you meditate, this neural connection between the center of your bodily sensation and your "Me" center is weakened. This means that you don't react as strongly to sensations that might have once stimulated your "Me" Center.

Interestingly, as this connection between the "Me" center and the center of your bodily sensation is weakened, the neural connections between what's known as your Assessment Center (Lateral prefrontal cortex) and the center of your bodily sensation and fear center are strengthened simultaneously. The Assessment center is that part of the brain that allows you to look at things from a more rational, logical and balanced perspective. This part of your brain is known for reasoning and it is involved in modulating emotional responses originating from the fear center (amygdala) or other parts of the brain, overriding automatic behaviors or habits and decreasing the brain's tendency to take things personally (by modulating the Me Center of the brain). So when you experience a scary or upsetting sensation, you can more easily look at them rationally.

For example, when you experience pain, rather than becoming anxious and assuming it means something is wrong with you, you can watch the pain rise and fall without becoming ensnared in a story about what it might mean. So there is less or no anxiety.

Deactivating the "Me" Center makes us Happier

One of the most interesting studies in the last few years, carried out at Yale University, found that mindfulness meditation decreases activity in the default mode network (DMN), also called the "Me" Center, comprising of the brain network responsible for mind-wandering and self-referential thoughts. The DMN is "on" or active when we're not thinking about anything in particular, when our minds are just wandering from thought to thought. Since mind-wandering is typically associated with being less happy, ruminating, and worrying about the past and future, you need to reduce it to feel happier. Several studies have shown that meditation, through its quieting effect on the DMN, appears to do just that. And even when the mind does start to wander, because of the new connections that form, meditators are better at snapping back out of this habit.

Meditation Chronic Stress and Relaxation Response:

In chronic stress there is a perpetually increased level of stress hormones. Chronic stress leads sooner or later to what is usually called a 'burnout'. It manifests as psychological and physiological disturbances and ultimately diseases. The symptoms may include psychosomatic disorders (e.g. tensed neck, headache, gastritis and irritable bowel), pronounced tiredness, low psychological endurance and concentration ability, memory disturbances, inner tensions, anxiety, sleep disturbances and depression. But before these symptoms, people may have a high stress hormone level for years without being aware of being "stressed".

There is a connection between chronically increased levels of stress hormones and the so called "metabolic syndrome" that appears as increased abdominal fat, increased blood lipids, tendency for high blood pressure and a tendency for diabetes. This syndrome brings about a significantly increased risk for atherosclerotic cardiovascular disease including stroke, angina pectoris and myocardial infarction.

In 1970s Harvard cardiologist Harvard Benson (Benson, Beary, and Carol 1974) found that practitioners of Transcendental meditation show a constellation of physiological changes suggesting deepened relaxation. These include as we've discussed earlier— reduced heart rate, blood pressure, brainwave activity, respiratory rate and so on. Dr. Benson's research popularized the definition of relaxation as Generalized Reduced Arousal and Relaxation Response. Relaxation response is just the mirror image of Stress response. During the stress sympathetic nervous system becomes dominant whereas during relaxation response the parasympathetic nervous system plays a dominant role.

Dr. Benson's Studies showed that meditation Induced following Relaxation Responses:

- Metabolism decreases

- Muscles relax

- Heart beats slower

- Blood pressure decreases

- Levels of Nitric Oxide in the body increases

These findings have been confirmed by other studies: Rai et al. 1988; Young & Taylor 2001.

Serotonin and Relaxation Response

Serotonin is an important signal mediator in the nervous system. Higher levels are associated with a relaxed and pleasant mood. Animal experiments indicate that lowered levels of serotonin are related to a chronic increase of the stress hormone cortisol (Sapolsky RM 1992, Sapolsky RM 1984). Several observations indicate that the same may be true for humans. It has been found that the levels of cortisol are decreased when precursors to serotonin are given to a subject (Maes M et al 1990). Increased levels of stress hormone cortisol have also been demonstrated in psychoses, panic syndrome, and anorexia nervosa. In all these conditions the serotonin levels have been found to be low.

How Anxiety can Become Chronic

Serotonin inhibits the activity in a part of the brain called Locus Coeruleus (LC) (Aston-Jones G 1991). Increased activity in LC is associated with feelings of anxiety, anger, fear and frustration. As stress lowers the Serotonin levels, the activity in LC is increased (Nisenbaum LK 1991).

It leads to a vicious circle of anxiety chain as follows:

anxiety-> Stress-> increased cortisol-> low tryptophan level (Tryptophan is a precursor to Serotonin) -> decreased Serotonin production-> low Serotonin level -> increased LC activity-> more Anxiety and stress.

This cycle goes on perpetually reinforcing the stress condition leading to chronic stress or anxiety, which may create many more neurological or psychological disorder in the long run.

How can Transcendental Meditation Lower Chronic Stress

TM has been found to lower the cortisol level. The lowering is greater in those who practice TM regularly. Both these effect are more pronounced in advanced practitioners (Jevning R et al. 1992, Jevning R et al 1978) (Jevning, Wallace, and Beidebach 1992). Also, the serotonin levels have been found to increase during TM (Bujatti M, Riederer P, 1976). Regular practice is thus likely to increase the average serotonin level. Thus the level of stress decreases naturally.

Clinical Application of Relaxation Response

A randomized clinical trial by Dr. Jane Leserman and colleagues, including Dr. Benson from the Harvard medical school studied twenty seven patients undergoing cardiac surgery. The meditation method they used in the study is called the Relaxation Response. The patients in the group randomized to practice meditation had a statistically significant lower incidence of tachycardia syndrome called supraventricular tachycardia compared to the control group. Another clinical trial led by Dr. Benson published in the journal Lancet studied patients with coronary artery disease who practiced the relaxation response for twenty minutes twice daily. After four weeks, a reduced frequency of the dysrhythmia called premature ventricular contractions (PVCs) was documented in eight of eleven patients studied.

In his book 'The Healing Power of Meditation: Your Prescription for Getting Well and Staying Well With Meditation', Dr. Gabriel Weiss says that meditation techniques can be effective means for treating some of the heart rhythm problems. In his book he relates the case of one of his patients Jim, who was a semi-retired former police officer. Even after his retirement Jim continued his consulting work in disaster management. Jim had a past history of bypass surgery and was taking beta-blocker medicine for his blood pressure. Jim came to see Dr. Weiss when he was experiencing a feeling of faster heartbeat (that is, tachycardia) and a sensation of palpitation associated with an irregular pulse. He had recently received an offer to work on a big project in Japan to provide his consultancy on disaster preparedness.

When he came to his doctor's office, Jim looked a little anxious, but his physical exam was almost normal, according to Dr. Weiss, except for a slightly elevated Blood pressure and an electrocardiogram revealed an occasional PVC, but was otherwise normal. Dr. Weiss ordered a screening cardiac stress test, which also turned out normal. Dr. Weiss then recommended Jim to try meditation to reduce his stress and see if it would help reduce his blood pressure and palpitations.

Following his doctor's instruction, Jim started coming in meditation classes and learned a breath meditation. Dr. Weiss's observation was: He took to meditation as a duck takes to water. Subsequent tests revealed that his palpitations and PVCs stopped, and his blood pressure returned to normal. He happily went ahead with his new professional responsibility.

This was a doctor's firsthand account on how he prescribed meditation, taught it, and witnessed his patients healed by this.

In his book, Dr. Weiss talks about Rick, another patient, who is a doctor himself, a retired dermatologist. After retirement Rick found interest in many branches of alternative medicines, including herbal medicine. Dr. Rick had a high cholesterol level, but he was afraid of the possible side effects of Statin drugs that are usually prescribed to treat high cholesterol. He instead started taking herbal supplements, which unfortunately did not work to lower his cholesterol. Rick also had occasional vague feelings of chest discomfort, which they later found out due to recurrent episodes of angina.

Rick started coming to the meditation classes and overcame his fear for medication. He subsequently underwent bypass surgery and now leading an active life with meditation.

Chapter Ten

Meditation and Brain Fitness

Brain fitness is the ability of a human being to meet efficiently the diverse cognitive demands of everyday life. It includes the ability to assimilate information, understand relationships, and develop reasonable conclusions and plans. Scientific research confirmed that meditation along with sound sleep, healthy lifestyle, mental stimulation, physical exercise and good nutrition can improve brain fitness.

Adverse Impact of Stress on Brain: How Meditation Can Help

Chronic stress, anxiety and depression can decrease brain fitness. The brain is one of the most vulnerable targets for stress and stress-related hormones. It undergoes functional and structural remodeling in response to stress, and can lead to damage when stress is excessive (McEwen and Morrison 2013). Chronic stress increases the stress hormone cortisol and adversely affects many brain functions. The stress hormone cortisol creates a surplus of the neurotransmitter glutamate (Bremner 2006), which generates free radicals, unattached oxygen molecules that attack brain cells punching holes in the brain cell walls, causing the cells to rupture and die (Alekseenko et al. 2010). Memory problems may be one of the first signs of stress you'll notice. In a recent study, chronic stress was shown to impair learning and memory functions (Kim and Leem 2016). Stress causes loss in brain cells everyday, but there is the opportunity to grow new ones. Brain-derived neurotrophic factor (BDNF) is a protein that is vital for the growth of new brain cells and keeping existing brain cells healthy. BDNF can offset the negative effects of stress on the brain. But cortisol reduces the production of BDNF resulting in fewer new brain cells being formed. Thus, high level of oxidative stress may eventually give rise to accumulation of oxidative damage and development of numerous neurodegenerative diseases. It has been presented that brain-derived neurotrophic factor (BDNF) supports neurons against various neurodegenerative conditions. Lowered levels of BDNF, as found in chronic stress conditions, are associated with brain-related conditions including depression, schizophrenia, dementia, and Alzheimer's disease (Yang et al. 2015). Meditation, specially, mindfulness meditation has been shown to reduce stress (Tang, Hölzel, and Posner 2015). Research over the past two decades largely supports the claim that mindfulness meditation — practiced generally for the reduction of stress and promotion of health — exerts beneficial effects on physical and mental health, and cognitive performance. Recent neuroimaging studies have begun to uncover the brain areas and networks that mediate these positive effects. Some forms of mindfulness meditation training have been found to reduce stress-induced cortisol secretion, which could potentially have neuro-protective effects by increasing levels of BDNF.

Impact of Meditation on Different Brain Areas

Mindfulness meditation has been seen to benefit the brain significantly, thereby improving executive and decision making functions, increasing cortical thickness, increasing attention and motivation. The Impact of meditation on brain has been seen as follows. Research highlights on Mindfulness based practices in clinical settings:

Brain Region		Observation
1.	Dorsolateral prefrontal cortex(dlPFC) is activated consistently	- Improved Executive decision making functions; Increased cortical Thickness
2.	Anterior Cingulate Cortex(ACC) is also activated	- Integrated attention, motivation and motor control
3.	Insula is activated	- Associated with pain control, emotion control and "gut feeling"
4.	Increased cortical thickness in Prefrontal cortex, anterior	- Noticed in long-term meditators; may lead to better decision making

Professor Richardson and his colleagues reported that the left and right prefrontal cortex (PFC) play differential roles in emotional processing. They have shown that stimulated positive and negative affective states shift the symmetry in prefrontal brain electrical activity; negative effect increases relative right-sided activation whereas positive effect increases relative left-sided activation. They have observed that meditation increases the left-sided activation.

How Meditation Changes the Brain Structure

Until 1970s the prevailing scientific view was that the brain remains static once we reach adulthood, that its functioning remains the same. Since then neuroscience has progressed a lot and came to know about 'Neuroplasticity', which means that the brain continues to form new neural connection throughout our lives.

All experiences in terms of what we feel, sense and think can change the brain's physical structure and its functional organization. It follows therefore that the more we practice something as any type of meditation, corresponding changes will take place in the brain.

Modern technologies such as FMRI (Functional Magnetic Resonance imaging) and EEG (Electroencephalography) makes it possible for the neuroscientists to see exactly what goes on in the brain when we meditate, and these are being used to understand the effect of meditation.

Thus modern studies shed light on how continued practice leads to lasting changes in the brain.

Researchers at UCLA wanted to study the brains of experienced meditators – people who had been meditating for years, versus those who had never meditated or who had only done it for a short period of time. They took MRI scans of 100 people — half of them were meditators and half, non-meditators. Researchers were fascinated to find that long-time meditators showed higher levels of gyrification (a folding of the cerebral cortex that may be associated with faster information processing and higher intelligence). In a study published in Frontiers in Human Neuroscience in February of 2012, they shared that the more years a person had been meditating, the more gyrification their MRIs revealed.

Meditation May Lead to Volume Changes in Key Areas of the Brain

In 2011, Sara Lazar (Hölzel et al. 2011) and her team at Harvard found that mindfulness meditation can actually change the brain structure. Eight weeks of Mindfulness-Based Stress Reduction (MBSR) was reported to increase cortical thickness in the hippocampus, which governs learning and memory, and in certain areas of the brain that play roles in emotion regulation, empathy and self-referential processing.

They also noticed decreases in brain cell volume in the amygdala, which is responsible for fear, anxiety, and stress. These changes in brain structure matched the participants' self-reports of their stress levels, indicating that meditation not only changes the brain, but it changes our subjective perception and feelings as well.

A follow-up study by Lazar's (Singleton et al. 2014) team found that after meditation training, changes in brain areas linked to mood and arousal were also linked to improvements in how participants reported about their feelings — i.e., their psychological well-being.

Meditation Strengthens the Prefrontal Cortex

Prefrontal cortex (PFC) is the cerebral cortex which covers the front part of the brain. The frontal lobes, located in the forehead, are the most front area of the brain. The most important portion of this area is called the pre-frontal cortex. This is the most evolved part of the human brain.

Meditation and Brainwaves

EEG findings arising from different types of meditation has shown

- Higher basal levels of Alpha and Theta band activity(associated with restful awareness and sleep)

- More consistent increase with theta band activity (Associated with sleep)

- Different meditation techniques elicited different patterns of brain activity (Lehman et al,2001)

Meditation techniques that emphasize deep physical relaxation produce higher theta (4-7Hz) and delta (1-4 Hz.) activity.

Beta level is associated with ordinary conversation and rational thinking in waking state. And emission of Theta characterizes a sleepy state or dream state and delta is deep sleep.

Does Meditation Increase Creativity?

More intense concentration and mindfulness meditation produces higher Alpha (8-12Hz.) activity. Emission of Alpha brainwave is associated with increased creativity and focus. Scientists, poets and artists are known to exist in Alpha state when they do their work.

Researchers at Leiden University in the Netherlands looked at two types of meditation — focused-attention (for example, focusing on your breath) and open-monitoring (where participants focus on the both the internal and external) — to find out how they affected creative thinking — the ability to generate new ideas and solutions to problems. In a study, Lorenza et al. (Colzato, Ozturk, and Hommel 2012) published in April 2012 in Frontiers in Cognition, reported that the participants who practiced focused-attention meditation did not show improved results in the two types creativity tasks. However, those who practiced open-monitoring meditation performed better at task related to coming up with new ideas. Indeed, the two types of meditation affected the two types of thinking in opposite ways: while convergent thinking tended to improve after focused attention meditation and divergent thinking was significantly enhanced after open monitoring meditation. Similarly, some other studies support a strong positive impact of meditation practice on creativity (Lippelt, Hommel, and Colzato 2014).

Mind Body Connection

In the olden day medical science used to draw stark line of demarcation between the body and mind, between physical and mental health. Even now those two were considered two distinctly separate disciplines.

But modern research has documented something very interesting. Mind does and can alter the state of the physiological functioning of the body.

An interesting study on meditation was conducted on sight in the sub-zero degrees of the Himalayas, where Dr. Benson and his colleagues studied Tibetan monks who, through controlling autonomic process, were able to voluntarily generate enough body-heat to produce steam and eventually dry the wet sheets draped around their bodies. While they documented the remarkable physiological feat of the Tibetan monks, Benson Lehman et al (1982)(BENSON, HERBERT, LEHMANN, JOHN,

MALHOTRA, W.M. S. , GOLDMAN 1982)(Kozhevnikov et al. 2013) succeeded in confirming the mind-body connection beyond doubt.

Neuro-Biological Impact of Meditation

Meditation, specially open monitoring and compassion meditation induces what one may consider a low-entropy state of equanimous, vigilant awareness, bringing the body to a hypo-metabolic state of parasympathetic dominance that serves to rejuvenate the organism's capacity for resilience and adaptability.

Chapter Eleven

Meditation and Default Mode Network

Our brain has large scale neural networks called Intrinsic Connectivity Networks (ICN) that may function either in an active mode or in a passive or resting state. Scientists have found two temporarily distinct functional networks.

1) CEN or Central executive network also called the Task positive network (TPN). Momentary self reference centered on present moment, called experiential focus, is neurologically connected with central executive network. This network is activated during when our attention is focused.

2) DMN or Default mode network. Extended self reference linking subjective experience across time is neurologically correlated with Default mode network. Default mode network is generally active when one is idle and its function is characterized by ruminative, often subconscious self

referential narrative thoughts, which generates our concept of self or identity. DMN becomes activated in the absence of focused mental tasks. Conversely CEN is activated and DMN deactivated during focused mental tasks.

Another related ICN of importance to overall health and mental wellbeing is Salience Network associated with resilience and perseverance in the face of stress. The salience network (SN) is known to act as a sort of frequency modulator between the activation of the CEN in the face of cognitively demanding task, and the simultaneous deactivation of the DMN.

Default mode network came to light when Dr. Marcus Raichle, a neurologist at the Washington University School of Medicine in the US State of Missouri, began scanning the brain of individuals who were not given any task to perform. The patients quickly became bored, and Dr. Raichle noticed a second network, that had previously gone unnoticed, danced with activity.

Default mode network has been deeply placed under the focus of scientific observation in the recent years, because, it is believed that a hyperactive Default mode network is the cause of many neurological disorders. Scientists previously believed that the self-reflective DMN in the brain was simply one that was active when a person had no task to focus their attention on. But researchers have found in the past decade that this section of the brain swells with activity when the subject thinks about self.

Another interesting fact emerged when the scientists subjected some Tibetan monks under experiment during their meditation. Neuroscientist Dr. Josipovic found that some Buddhist monks and experienced meditators have the ability to keep both the neural networks— CEN and DMN— active at the same time during their meditation. This was something startling, to say the least, because, CEN and DMN were thought to be rarely fully active at the same time. Like a seesaw, when one rises the other goes down. But the meditators were achieving this abnormal feat of keeping both the regions active at the same time! Some neuro scientists believe that this has something to do with their feelings of oneness and tranquility. This finding also proved that there are two aspects of DMN. One is meditative self absorbed state, and the second one is mind wandering and constantly chattering obsessive thinking or ego-centric rumination.

Now scientists believe that through Self-aware focus in meditation a balance between the two networks can be established that can generate a feeling of serenity and wellbeing, keeping the meditators mentally healthy.

Now abnormal activity in the ICN has been implicated in a number of psychiatric diseases e.g., ADHD, Bipolar disorder, Borderline personality disorder, depression, Anxiety disorder and Schizophrenia. An inability to switch off the hyperactive Default Mode Network through focused attention appears to be major contributor in these disease processes.

Now recent findings have proved that a gradual meditation induced functional reorganization of brainwave patterns takes place between the DMN, SN and CEN, where reliance upon DMN seems to decrease and reliance on CEN and SN seems to increase. Now scientists are saying that since DMN seems to be a major network in the brain that seems to be very much involved in a lot of neurological disorders, including autism and Alzheimer's, reducing reliance on DMN through focused attention in meditation can be helpful in preventing diseases like Alzheimer's; because meditation in general reduces the activities of the DMN.

Meditation has been associated with relatively reduced activity in the default mode network (Garrison et al. 2015). Meditators also reported significantly less mind-wandering, which are normally associated with activity in the DMN. Researchers also found that the main nodes of the default-mode network (medial prefrontal and posterior cingulate cortices) were relatively deactivated in experienced meditators across all meditation types; concentration meditation, Loving-Kindness meditation and choiceless awareness meditation (Brewer et al. 2011). Studies have also suggest that meditation training leads to functional connectivity changes between core DMN regions (Taylor et al. 2013). They observed that relative to beginners, experienced meditators have weaker functional connectivity between DMN regions that involved in self-referential processing and emotional appraisal.

Chapter Twelve

Meditation and Longevity: Does Meditation Slow Down Aging?

In the olden times people lived a life synchronized with the Nature, and many of them lived a full life, happy, healthy and stress-free. My own granny lived up to 97 years. I have seen people living their 100th year, disease-free, medication-free! Then how come our present society is burdened so much with disease and medication? Where did we lose the track? What went wrong with us?

In olden times people lived a naturally meditative life, close to a natural setting. Meditative practices like contentment and letting go was a way of life. In modern age of consumerism and social networking, restlessness, agitation, feverish goal-setting and desire has been the common norm. Hence, to get respite from this type of stressed lifestyle, the need for having a practice of meditation has become more relevant in modern times than any other ages.

As we have seen, meditation training seems to protect against stress and boosts the immune system. It has also recently been shown to reduce neuronal decay due to normal aging. Pagnoni and Cekic (2007) found greater prefrontal cortex thickness in middle-aged meditators than in non-meditators, as well as a decline in cortical thickness associated with age, a result that is also reported by Lazar et al. (2005) (Lazar et al. 2005).

Age is negatively associated with gray matter volume. Elderly people show lower volumes of gray matters in the brain. Gray matters are directly linked to memory and reduction of gray matters causes memory problems for elderly people. Recent research has proved that mindfulness meditation is a simple way to increases gray matter volume in the brain.

Nagendra, Sulekha, Tubaki, and Kutty (2008) also showed that expert Vipassana meditators did not present sleep patterns associated with aging. Both the length of the slow waves sleep period before the occurrence of the first REM sleep episode and the total length of REM episodes typically decrease with age. They showed that this decrease was drastically smaller in meditators of age 50–60 than in control subjects of the same age. This suggests that meditation slows down the brain-aging process.

Loving Kindness Meditation Slows Down Aging

Stress decreases telomere length, which are a biological marker of aging. Hoge et al (2013) (Hoge et al. 2013) found that women with experience in Loving Kindness Meditation had relatively longer telomere length compared to age-matched controls.

Seven Health Benefits of Deep Relaxation induced by meditation Associated with delayed Aging:

1. Increased Immunity: A study at the Ohio State University found that deep relaxation techniques when practiced daily boost natural killer cells (NKC) in the elderly giving them greater resistance to tumor and viruses.

2. Greater Emotional balance: Emotional balance means to be free from all neurotic behavior that results from the existence of a tortured and traumatized ego that carries the burden of many past impressions and consistently is colored by emotionally soaked memories making a person unable to make a neutral and appropriate response to a present event. As people grow older, they normally carry many burdens of past hurt, resentment and unhappy memory; that makes many elderly people grumpy, easily irritable, and complaining type. Older people often feel disconnected from the world. Meditation facilitates letting go of the past, and helps us stay in the present. Meditation has been

proved to endow people with greater emotional balance, clarity, enthusiasm and patience. That is reversal of aging, so far as a person's behavior or view of the world is concerned. Especially, the loving Kindness meditation helps people to become more empathetic and socially connected.

3. Meditation is Anti-inflammatory. Elderly people are often subject to inflammatory diseases, e.g., heart disease, arthritis and the like. Stress leads to inflammation, a state linked to heart disease, arthritis, Asthma and skin conditions such as psoriasis, says researchers at Emory University in the US. Meditation can help prevent and treat such symptoms by switching off the stress response.

4. Loss of brain volume is a symptom associated with aging. Meditation has been found to increase grey matter, increase cerebral plasticity and cerebral blood flow, as well as thickness in the brain regions.

6. Normally elderly people have disturbed sleep pattern. Meditation has been proved to improve sleep pattern. Practitioners of TM

and Loving Kindness meditation are known to sleep well.

7. Increase in GABA is another positive effect of meditation that can reverse aging.

Chapter Thirteen

Research in Loving Kindness Meditation

Research shows that Loving Kindness Meditation has a tremendous amount of benefits ranging from benefitting well-being, to giving relief from illness and improving emotional intelligence.

Loving Kindness meditation increases wellbeing and positive emotions

Researcher Barbara Fredrickson at the University of North Carolina at Chapel Hill took working adults and assigned them randomly to a loving kindness meditation group or to a control group. In this landmark study, Barbara Frederickson(Fredrickson et al. 2008) and her colleagues found that practicing 7 weeks of loving-kindness meditation increased love, joy, contentment, gratitude, pride, hope, interest, amusement, and awe. Dr. Fredrickson and her team investigated the impact of LKM not only on emotions, but also on how this practice could actually build personal resources (cognitive, emotional, and physical).

They found that these positive emotions then produced increases in a wide range of personal resources, including increased mindful attention, self-acceptance, purpose in life, social support, positive relationships with others, decreased illness symptoms and good physical health. Ultimately, these personal resources enabled people to become more satisfied with their lives and to experience fewer symptoms of depression. These findings are powerful.

Loving Kindness Meditation Increases Vagal Tone

Loving kindness meditation is also known to increase vagal tone which increases positive emotions & feelings of social connection. A study by Kok et al (2013) (Kok et al. 2013) found that individuals in a Loving Kindness Meditation intervention, compared to a control group, had increases in positive emotions, an effect moderated by baseline vagal tone – a physiological marker of well-being.

Loving Kindness Meditation Decreases Migraines

A recent study by Tonelli et al (2014) (Tonelli and Wachholtz 2014) demonstrated the immediate effects of a brief Loving Kindness Meditation intervention in reducing migraine pain and alleviating emotional tension associated with chronic migraines.

Twenty-seven migraine patients, with two to ten migraines per month, reported the effect on migraine-related pain and emotional tension before and after exposure to a brief meditation-based treatment. All participants were meditation- naïve, and attended one 20 minute guided meditation session based on the Buddhist "loving kindness" approach. After the session, participants reported a 33% decrease in pain and a 43% decrease in emotional tension. The researchers concluded that just a single exposure to a brief meditative technique could significantly reduce pain and tension.

Loving Kindness Meditation Decreases Chronic Pain

A Duke University Medical Center pilot study tested an eight-week loving kindness program for chronic low back pain patients. In this pilot study of patients with chronic lower back pain, where the patients were randomly exposed to Loving Kindness Meditation or standard care, Carson[6] et al. found that Loving Kindness Meditation was associated with greater decrease in pain, anger and psychological distress than the control group.

Loving Kindness Meditation Decreases PTSD

A study by Kearney et al. in 2013 (Kearney et al. 2013) found that a 12 week Loving Kindness Meditation course significantly reduced depression and PTSD symptoms among veterans diagnosed with PTSD.

Loving Kindness Meditation Decreases Schizophrenia-Spectrum Disorders

Another pilot study by Johnson et al. in 2011 (Johnson et al. 2011) examining the effects of Loving Kindness Meditation with individuals with schizophrenia-spectrum disorders, found that Loving Kindness Meditation was associated with decreased negative symptoms and increased positive emotions and psychological recovery.

Loving Kindness Meditation Increases Respiratory Sinus Arrythmia

Respiration rate is correlated with psychological well-being. In particular, chronic rapid, irregular breathing patterns are associated with increased anxiety as well as clinical pain and anxiety disorders. Conversely, controlled breathing, especially deep, slow breathing, is established as an effective short-term intervention in behavioral health settings, and has been shown to reduce autonomic reactivity, negative mood, and pain-related distress

(Wielgosz et al. 2016). Just 10 minutes of loving-kindness meditation has an immediate relaxing effect as evidenced by increased respiratory sinus arrhythmia (RSA), and slowed (i.e. more relaxed) respiration rate (Law 2012).

Loving Kindness Meditation Increases Empathy and Positive Mental States

Neuroimaging studies suggest that Loving Kindness Meditation and Compassion Meditation may enhance activation of brain areas that are involved in emotional processing and empathy.

Studies by and Hutcherson, Seppala & Gross, (Seppala et al. 2014) showed that regularly practicing loving-kindness meditation activates and strengthens areas of the brain responsible for empathy & emotional intelligence.

Loving Kindness Meditation has also seen to increase relaxation, decrease stress response, increase social connection, increase empathetic behavior, improve self image and decrease self criticism.

Loving Kindness Meditation Increases Telomere length – a biological marker of aging

Stress decreases telomere length (telomeres are tiny bits of chromosomes, your genetic material. Telomeres are a biological marker of aging. Relatively short telomere length may serve as a marker of accelerated aging, and shorter telomeres have been connected to chronic stress. Hoge et al (Hoge et al. 2013) found that women with experience in Loving Kindness Meditation had relatively longer telomere length compared to age-matched controls.

Chapter Fourteen

Reap the Benefit Now: How to Meditate

We have come to the last phase of our journey. By now I hope you are convinced that meditation can do us a whole lot of good. We all know that meditation can benefit us, physically, mentally and spiritually. But, how many of us meditate everyday? Off course, I know many of my esteemed readers will say that you are too busy to find a time to meditate, because you have many duties and responsibilities to attend to.

That is true, I know. But meditation is a duty to yourself, and unless you do this duty to yourself, your other duties can not be performed with full efficiency. Meditation is the process of charging your own battery. Believe me, it is not lack of time that make people postpone meditation. It is a question of habit. If you have time to enjoy a cup of tea, you have time to meditate. If you can breathe, you can meditate. It is as simple as that. Begin with a small dose, as little as 5 minutes a day, and increase it to at least 15 minutes.

When to Meditate and How Long to Meditate

Meditate any time morning or evening. If possible, schedule a set time to practice each day. Set aside one or two periods each day. You may find that it's easier to stick with your practice. You can do meditation in the morning. For beginners 5 to 10 minutes of meditation is good enough. You may increase that gradually to fifteen minutes to forty minutes. Gradually, you'll find a knack of it, and you may naturally want to meditate for a longer session.

How to Meditate: A Simple Breath Meditation that can Transform your Life

Prepare to meditate by finding a quiet room without distractions and take the following steps. Turn off your phone and any other gadgets. Dim the lights and play soothing music if you like. The point is to create an environment conducive to freeing your mind from its daily clutter and relaxing your body.

Step 1: Sit comfortably and decide how long you want to meditate

You can sit on the floor, on a chair, in your car or any place where you are comfortable. Beginners often struggle to find the best posture for meditation. Actually there's no "right" way to meditate. Only thing you need to remember is that your spine should be straight, and you should not slump during meditation. Keep your back straight so you can breathe deeply with ease.

Sit on the floor, If you can, and close your eyes. You don't have to sit in the lotus position unless you want to, but sitting on the floor helps you feel grounded, and it connects you to Mother Earth. Feel free to use pillows or cushions that help you feel comfortable. If sitting on the floor is too uncomfortable, sit in a straight-backed chair with your head forward, knees bent at right angle and your hands on your thighs, and place your feet firmly on the floor to develop a sense of grounding.

Keep your eyes half opened, or closed, whichever way you feel comfortable. Keeping your eyes closed minimize the distractions for the beginners.

Then decide how long you want to meditate today. I suggest you to commit a shorter period, say 8 minutes, if you are a beginner. You may set a timer for this purpose.

Step 2: Enjoy your breathing

Comfortably, fill up the whole of your lungs with air. Breathe in and out slowly through your nose for 5 times.

Step 3: Honour your feelings

Watch and accept your feelings.

Step 4: Observe your Breathing

Focus your attention at the gate of your nostrils and feel the sensation of breathing. Feel the air coming in, and going out of your nostrils. Notice the process of your natural breathing, without interfering with it. Do not try to control anything.

Now mentally note "In", when the air comes in, and "Out", when the air goes out. Stay with your normal breathing this way. Do not try to alter anything. If your breathing is shallow, or uneven, let it be so. If your breathing eventually becomes deep, let it be so. If your breathing is rugged, let it be so; if it is soft and smooth, let it be so. Just be like a gatekeeper and put your attention at the gate of your nostrils, and go on mentally making a note of it, when the breath enters your nostrils, and when it leaves your nostrils.

Initially, you'll find your attention wander away for several times to thoughts, mental images, and daily trivia. Whenever you catch your mind going away from breath, just bring it back to breath with a smile. Know that this is perfectly normal, and even the Buddha had to face such mind-wandering when he didn't attain to Buddhahood!

Just persistently stick to the process of watching your breath, and bringing your attention back to your breath, if it wanders to something else. Do it for the specific period of time, you decided to do, until the timer goes out.

Step 5: Let go of your thoughts and don't judge

Negative thoughts and feelings may pop up, during the process. Allow them to go with a long outgoing breath. Just focus on the present moment. Accept your natural feelings without judgment of good or bad. Staying with your breath is the most important thing, for the moment. Gently bring your attention back to your natural breathing.

Not judging yourself is most important when you learn to meditate. Criticizing yourself for a "bad" meditation session or beating yourself up because your chattering mind won't calm you down. Remain compassionate with yourself.

Closing the Meditation Session

When your meditation is over, smile and congratulate yourself for being able to do it anyway. Thank your body for cooperating with you. Thank your mind for having patience during the session. Thank the earth for supporting you. Thank the cosmos, and all the beneficial forces and beings that might have helped your meditation with or without your conscious knowledge.

Now wish for the good of all. Wish for the well being of yourself. Wish for the well being of your family. Wish for the well being of others.

This deceptively simple meditation technique has been practiced since ages, and was made popular by the Buddha, who practiced it himself for reaching stages of enlightenment. This meditation brings us home to the peace of present-moment awareness. It gives us a direct experience of the deeper peace that is buried within us, behind the constant chatter of the mind, and in the process dissolves the impurities which prevent the Spirit from shining forth in our lives.

This simple meditation, if practiced diligently, can transform the way you see the world and interact with others. It can change your perspective and make you a better human being. It has the potential to free you from anxiety, worry, and unhappiness, and make you calm, focused, poised and peaceful. Does it sound interesting? Then start doing it from today. Like anything, it just takes practice. With regular practice, it really does get easier, and the benefits are so worth the effort.

Mantra Meditation: An Age-old Practice for Stress Reduction

Mantra meditation is an age-old practice for quieting the mind. During the meditation, you need not forcing your mind to be quiet; instead you experience the silence and stillness that lies beyond the background static of worry, resentment, wishful thinking, fantasy, unfulfilled desires, and cobwebs of dreams in your head.

In this meditation we disrupt the unconscious progression of thoughts and emotions by focusing on a new object of attention. In this meditation technique we the "object of attention" is a mantra that we repeat silently to ourselves. A mantra is pure sound, with no meaning or emotional charge to trigger associations. It allows the mind to detach from its usual preoccupations and experience the spaciousness and peace within.

You may pick up a mantra of your choice, one that resonates deeply within you, and silently repeat it in your mind, guiding your mind gently back to the mantra, when it wanders away. You can do it for ten to fifteen minutes, or as long you feel comfortable. One thing is very important in practicing this type of meditation. Never go on uttering your mantra unconsciously, while your mind runs with parallel stream of thoughts. Mentally utter the mantra distinctly, with brief pause before and after every utterance. As soon as you are aware that your mind has wandered, gently bring it back on the mantra.

Another important point to remember is that once you pick up a mantra, don't change it often. Stay with it for a considerable period of time.

Even more important than what you experience during your meditation sessions is the effect they have on the remaining hours of your day. With a regular practice of meditation, life's inevitable stressors no longer have the power to drown you into the turbulent ocean of chaotic mind-states; and all of your thoughts and actions will be infused with greater calmness, love, peace and joy.

A Healing Meditation involving Visualization

There are several different methods of meditative healing. A main form of healing meditation involves visualization. With visualization, some people imagine, or visualize, a white light running through their bodies and healing diseases or clearing their minds of stress or uncertainties. Healers often use the transfer of energy to heal diseases or physical conditions.

You can imagine a diseased internal organ bathed in light. Recently (Maureen 2010) in an interesting experiment Dr. William C. Bushell, an MIT-affiliated researcher in medical anthropology and NYU neuroscientist Dr. Zoran Josipovic placed a Tibetan Lama, Phakyab Rinpoche under a functional MRI scan, while he meditated inside the scanner at NYU's Center for Brain Imaging to examine his brain. This Lama claimed to cure his gangrene stricken leg by meditating for a year. The meditation he practiced is called Tsa Lung Meditation, which involved visualizing a wind (called 'lung' or 'Prana', that is one with the mind) moving down the center channel of his body, cleaning blockages and impurities, before moving on to even smaller channels. This cognitive behavioral practice, according to Dr. Bushell, may be "more effective than any strictly western medical intervention". They predicted that during the meditation practice, the Lama's body underwent mild to moderate hyperthermia, which might have killed the bacteria responsible for gangrene, and aided the body in healing.

Dr. Bushell and Dr. Josipovic's experiment bears testimony to earlier research findings that shows that mental imagery directed to sites of the body, both superficial as well as deeper tissues, can, with practice, lead to increased local blood flow, metabolic activity and oxygenation. Such increases could combat even powerful bacteria like Staphylococcus Aureus, which might be cause of Gangrene.

Start Meditation Today!

Stress is the worst enemy of modern high paced living. The stress hormone Cortisol is the most dangerous chemical to deal with. Meditation gives you the weapon to deal with them. Meditation is an Ancient Art of relaxation, Self-Healing and self realization.

This book in your hand can be an important asset for you if it encourages and inspires you to start meditation, or stick to it, if you are already in the practice.

Do not postpone meditation anymore. It can be the greatest and most beautiful gift you can give to yourself. Start it today. It is not difficult at all. Just observe your breath - one breath at a time. Sit quietly. Be with **your** breathing, and soon you will be meditating.

Chapter Fifteen

Conclusion and Future Scope

In this contribution we have focused on four classical areas of meditation research: meditation for brain fitness, meditation for cardiovascular health, meditation for immunity and meditation as an anti aging tool. There are various types of meditations. However, mindfulness meditation, transcendental meditation and loving kindness meditation seems to hold much promise as a way for preventing and curing stress related health problems.

The meditation research field seems to be getting into the maturing stage in its growing process where possibilities and the limits for preventing and curing diseases through meditation should be examined with more resources and more seriously. Despite the recent advances and the promise of more ahead, this young field still falls far short of a coherent picture of meditation mechanisms and effects. Meditation research requires collaborative and multidisciplinary research teams. Dynamic exchange of data, ideas and staff between the core clinical disciplines and other supportive disciplines are crucial for success. We believe that these types of collaborative and challenging research efforts will someday reveal much finer levels of clues about the effect of various meditation techniques on hormones, brain cells, neurotransmitters and DNA. In future, it will be possible to more systematically assess short- and long-term effects of meditation on different diseases.

But in general, so far researchers have not addressed the question of standardization of meditation techniques. Without standardization, it is not possible to understand the impact of finer levels of meditation techniques on individual. Some kind of benchmark for comparison must be developed.

The most important future area of research is large scale field tests which will determine whether anything useful comes out that significantly supports the preliminary exciting results. .Fundamental works on mathematical modeling and generalization of meditation techniques are required. That requires active participation of medical professionals, meditators and the researchers. Another major challenge is how to store, analyze, distribute, interpret, understand and use the enormous amount of data associated with every one of these thousands of images. Combining clinical data, imaging and molecular data in robust, extensible and distributed databases represents a fundamental need for modern meditation research. It is apparent that more methodologically rigorous studies are required if we are to gain full benefits of meditation for human well-being.

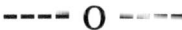 ---- O ----

References:

Alekseenko, A. V., V. A. Kolos, T. V. Waseem, and S. V. Fedorovich. 2010. "Glutamate Induces Formation of Free Radicals in Rat Brain Synaptosomes." *Biophysics* 54 (5): 617–20. doi:10.1134/S000635090905011X.

Benson, Herbert, John F. Beary, and Mark P. Carol. 1974. *The Relaxation Response. Psychiatry: Journal for the Study of Interpersonal Processes.* Vol. 37. http://psycnet.apa.org/psycinfo/1975-20469-001.

BENSON, HERBERT, LEHMANN, JOHN, MALHOTRA, W.M. S. , GOLDMAN, RALPH F. 1982. "Body Temperature Changes during the Practice of G Tum-Mo Yoga." *Nature* 295: 234–36. doi:doi:10.1038/295234a0.

Bono, J. 1984. "Psychological Assessment of Transcendental Meditation." In *Meditation: Classic and Contemporary Perspectives, Eds. D.H. Shapiro and R.N. Walsh.* New York: Aldine.

Bremner, J. Douglas. 2006. "Traumatic Stress: Effects on the Brain." *Dialogues in Clinical Neuroscience* 8 (4): 445–61.

Brewer, J. A., P. D. Worhunsky, J. R. Gray, Y.-Y. Tang, J. Weber, and H. Kober. 2011. "Meditation Experience Is Associated with Differences in Default Mode Network Activity and Connectivity." *Proceedings of the National Academy of Sciences* 108 (50): 20254–59. doi:10.1073/pnas.1112029108.

Colzato, Lorenza S., Ayca Ozturk, and Bernhard Hommel. 2012. "Meditate to Create: The Impact of Focused-Attention and Open-Monitoring Training on Convergent and Divergent Thinking." *Frontiers in Psychology* 3 (APR). doi:10.3389/fpsyg.2012.00116.

Davidson, Richard J, Jon Kabat-Zinn, Jessica Schumacher, Melissa Rosenkranz, Daniel Muller, Saki F Santorelli, Ferris Urbanowski, Anne Harrington, Katherine Bonus, and John F Sheridan. 2003. "Alterations in Brain and Immune Function Produced by Mindfulness Meditation." *Psychosomatic Medicine* 65 (4): 564–70. doi:10.1097/01.PSY.0000077505.67574.

E3.

Delmonte, M M. 1984. *Physiological Responses during Meditation and Rest. Biofeedback and Self-Regulation.* Vol. 9. doi:10.1007/BF00998833.

Engvig, Andreas, Anders M Fjell, Lars T Westlye, Torgeir Moberget, Øyvind Sundseth, Vivi Agnete Larsen, and Kristine B Walhovd. 2011. "Memory Training Impacts Short-Term Changes in Aging White Matter☐: A Longitudinal Diffusion Tensor Imaging Study" 00 (May). doi:10.1002/hbm.21370.

Epel, Elissa, Jennifer Daubenmier, Judith Tedlie Moskowitz, Susan Folkman, and Elizabeth Blackburn. 2009. "Can Meditation Slow Rate of Cellular Aging? Cognitive Stress, Mindfulness, and Telomeres." *Annals of the New York Academy of Sciences* 1172: 34–53. doi:10.1111/j.1749-6632.2009.04414.x.

Fredrickson, Barbara L, Michael a Cohn, Kimberly a Coffey, Jolynn Pek, and Sandra M Finkel. 2008. "Open Hearts Build Lives: Positive Emotions, Induced through Loving-Kindness Meditation, Build Consequential Personal

Resources." *Journal of Personality and Social Psychology* 95 (5): 1045–62. doi:10.1037/a0013262.

Garrison, Kathleen A., Thomas A. Zeffiro, Dustin Scheinost, Todd Constable, and Judson A. Brewer. 2015. "Meditation Leads to Reduced Default Mode Network Activity beyond an Active Task." *Cognitive Affective and Behavioral Neuroscience* 15: 712–20. doi:10.3758/s13415-015-0358-3.

Hofstetter, S, I Tavor, S Tzur Moryosef, and Y Assaf. 2013. "Short-Term Learning Induces White Matter Plasticity in the Fornix." *J Neurosci* 33 (31): 12844–50. doi:10.1523/jneurosci.4520 12.2013.

Hoge, Elizabeth a., Maxine M. Chen, Esther Orr, Christina a. Metcalf, Laura E. Fischer, Mark H. Pollack, Immaculata DeVivo, and Naomi M. Simon. 2013. "Loving-Kindness Meditation Practice Associated with Longer Telomeres in Women." *Brain, Behavior, and Immunity* 32: 159–63. doi:10.1016/j.bbi.2013.04.005.

Hölzel, Britta K, James Carmody, Mark Vangel, Christina Congleton, Sita M

Yerramsetti, Tim Gard, and Sara W Lazar. 2011. "Mindfulness Practice Leads to Increases in Regional Brain Gray Matter Density." *Psychiatry Research* 191 (1): 36–43. doi:10.1016/j.pscychresns.2010.08.006.

Jacobs, Tonya L., Elissa S. Epel, Jue Lin, Elizabeth H. Blackburn, Owen M. Wolkowitz, David a. Bridwell, Anthony P. Zanesco, et al. 2011. "Intensive Meditation Training, Immune Cell Telomerase Activity, and Psychological Mediators." *Psychoneuroendocrinology* 36. Elsevier Ltd: 664–81. doi:10.1016/j.psyneuen.2010.09.010.

Jevning, R, R K Wallace, and M Beidebach. 1992. "The Physiology of Meditation: A Review. A Wakeful Hypometabolic Integrated Response." *Neuroscience and Biobehavioral Reviews* 16 (57): 415–24. doi:10.1016/S0149-7634(05)80210-6.

Johnson, David P., David L. Penn, Barbara L. Fredrickson, Ann M. Kring, Piper S. Meyer, Lahnna I. Catalino, and Mary Brantley. 2011. "A Pilot Study of Loving-Kindness Meditation for the Negative Symptoms of Schizophrenia."

Schizophrenia Research 129 (2-3): 137–
40. doi:10.1016/j.schres.2011.02.015.

Kabat-Zinn J. 1990. *Full Catastrophy Living:
Using the Wisdom of Your Body and
Mind to Face Stress, Pain and Illness.*
New York: Dell Publishing.

Kearney, David J, Carol A Malte, Carolyn
Mcmanus, Michelle E Martinez, Ben
Felleman, and Tracy L Simpson. 2013.
"Loving-Kindness Meditation for
Posttraumatic Stress Disorder□: A Pilot
Study." *Journal of Traumatic Stress* 26
(August): 426–34. doi:10.1002/jts.

Kim, D-M, and Y-H Leem. 2016. "Chronic
Stress-Induced Memory Deficits Are
Reversed by Regular Exercise via AMPK-
Mediated BDNF Induction."
Neuroscience 324: 271–85.
doi:10.1016/j.neuroscience.2016.03.019.

Kok, Bethany E, Kimberly a Coffey, Michael a
Cohn, Lahnna I Catalino, Tanya
Vacharkulksemsuk, Sara B Algoe, Mary
Brantley, and Barbara L Fredrickson.
2013. "How Positive Emotions Build
Physical Health: Perceived Positive
Social Connections Account for the
Upward Spiral between Positive

Emotions and Vagal Tone."
Psychological Science 24 (7): 1123–32.
doi:10.1177/0956797612470827.

Kozhevnikov, Maria, James Elliott, Jennifer
Shephard, and Klaus Gramann. 2013.
"Neurocognitive and Somatic
Components of Temperature Increases
during G-Tummo Meditation: Legend
and Reality." *PloS One* 8 (3): e58244.
doi:10.1371/journal.pone.0058244.

Law, Rita W. 2012. "An Analogue Study of
Loving-Kindness Meditation as a Buffer
against Social Stress." *Dissertation
Abstracts International, B: Sciences and
Engineering* 72 (7): 4365.

Lazar, Sara W, Catherine E Kerr, Rachel H
Wasserman, Jeremy R Gray, Douglas N
Greve, Michael T Treadway, Metta
McGarvey, et al. 2005. "Meditation
Experience Is Associated with Increased
Cortical Thickness." *Neuroreport* 16 (17):
1893–97.

Lippelt, Dominique P., Bernhard Hommel,
and Lorenza S. Colzato. 2014. "Focused
Attention, Open Monitoring and Loving
Kindness Meditation: Effects on
Attention, Conflict Monitoring, and

Creativity - A Review." *Frontiers in Psychology* 5 (SEP). doi:10.3389/fpsyg.2014.01083.

Loh, Kep Kee, and Ryota Kanai. 2014. "Higher Media Multi-Tasking Activity Is Associated with Smaller Gray-Matter Density in the Anterior Cingulate Cortex." *PLoS ONE* 9 (9): e106698. doi:10.1371/journal.pone.0106698.

Maureen, Seaberg. 2010. *Can Meditation Cure Disease?* http://news.yahoo.com/meditation-cure-disease-20101225-161512-499.html.

McEwen, BruceS, and JohnH Morrison. 2013. "The Brain on Stress: Vulnerability and Plasticity of the Prefrontal Cortex over the Life Course." *Neuron* 79 (1): 16– 29. doi:10.1016/j.neuron.2013.06.028.

Olex, Stephen, Andrew Newberg, and Vincent M Figueredo. 2013. "Meditation: Should a Cardiologist Care?" *International Journal of Cardiology* 168 (3): 1805–10. doi:http://dx.doi.org/10.1016/j.ijcard.20 13.06.086.

Orme-Johnson, David W, Robert H Schneider, Young D Son, Sanford Nidich, and Zang-Hee Cho. 2006.

"Neuroimaging of Meditation's Effect on Brain Reactivity to Pain." *Neuroreport* 17 (12): 1359–63. doi:10.1097/01.wnr.0000233094.67289.a8.

Pace, Thaddeus W W, Lobsang Tenzin Negi, Daniel D. Adame, Steven P. Cole, Teresa I. Sivilli, Timothy D. Brown, Michael J. Issa, and Charles L. Raison. 2009. "Effect of Compassion Meditation on Neuroendocrine, Innate Immune and Behavioral Responses to Psychosocial Stress." *Psychoneuroendocrinology* 34 (1): 87–98. doi:10.1016/j.psyneuen.2008.08.011.

Paul-Labrador, M, D Polk, Dwyer JH, and et al. 2006. "EFfects of a Randomized Controlled Trial of Transcendental Meditation on Components of the Metabolic Syndrome in Subjects with Coronary Heart Disease." *Archives of Internal Medicine* 166 (11): 1218–24. http://dx.doi.org/10.1001/archinte.166.11.1218.

Pert, Candice. 2004. *The Molecules of Emotion*. New York.

Posner, Michael I., Yi Yuan Tang, and Gary

Lynch. 2014. "Mechanisms of White Matter Change Induced by Meditation Training." *Frontiers in Psychology* 5 (OCT). doi:10.3389/fpsyg.2014.01220.

Schneider, Robert H., Clarence E. Grim, Maxwell V. Rainforth, Theodore Kotchen, Sanford I. Nidich, Carolyn Gaylord-King, John W. Salerno, Jane Morley Kotchen, and Charles N. Alexander. 2012. "Stress Reduction in the Secondary Prevention of Cardiovascular Disease: Randomized, Controlled Trial of Transcendental Meditation and Health Education in Blacks." *Circulation: Cardiovascular Quality and Outcomes* 5 (6): 750–58. doi:10.1161/CIRCOUTCOMES.112.967406.

Seppala, Emma M, Cendri A Hutcherson, Dong T H Nguyen, James R Doty, and James J Gross. 2014. "Loving-Kindness Meditation: A Tool to Improve Healthcare Provider Compassion, Resilience, and Patient Care." *Journal of Compassionate Health Care* 1 (1): 1–9. doi:10.1186/s40639-014-0005-9.

Singleton, Omar, Britta K Hölzel, Mark

Vangel, Narayan Brach, James Carmody, and Sara W Lazar. 2014. "Change in Brainstem Gray Matter Concentration Following a Mindfulness-Based Intervention Is Correlated with Improvement in Psychological Well-Being." *Frontiers in Human Neuroscience* 8 (February): 33. doi:10.3389/fnhum.2014.00033.

Taimni, I.K. 1975. "Patanjali's 'Yoga Sutras' Book-I." In *In The Science of Yoga*, verses 2–4. Wheaton, IL: Theosophical Publishing House.

Tang, Yi-Yuan, Britta K Hölzel, and Michael I Posner. 2015. "The Neuroscience of Mindfulness Meditation." *Nature Reviews Neuroscience* 16 (4): 1–13. doi:10.1038/nrn3916.

Tanner, Melissa A., Fred Travis, Carolyn Gaylord-King, D. A F Haaga, Sarina Grosswald, and Robert H. Schneider. 2009. "The Effects of the Transcendental Meditation Program on Mindfulness." *Journal of Clinical Psychology* 65 (6): 574–89.

Taren, Adrienne A., Peter J. Gianaros, Carol M. Greco, Emily K. Lindsay, April

Fairgrieve, Kirk Warren Brown, Rhonda K. Rosen, et al. 2015. "Mindfulness Meditation Training Alters Stress-Related Amygdala Resting State Functional Connectivity: A Randomized Controlled Trial." *Social Cognitive and Affective Neuroscience* 10 (12): 1758–68. doi:10.1093/scan/nsv066.

Taylor, Véronique A., Véronique Daneault, Joshua Grant, Geneviève Scavone, Estelle Breton, Sébastien Roffe-vidal, Jérôme Courtemanche, et al. 2013. "Impact of Meditation Training on the Default Mode Network during a Restful State." *Social Cognitive and Affective Neuroscience* 8 (1): 4–14. doi:10.1093/scan/nsr087.

Tonelli, Makenzie E, and Amy B Wachholtz. 2014. "Meditation-Based Treatment Yielding Immediate Relief for Meditation-Naïve Migraineurs." *Pain Management Nursing□: Official Journal of the American Society of Pain Management Nurses* 15 (1): 36–40. doi:10.1016/j.pmn.2012.04.002.

Wielgosz, Joseph, Brianna S Schuyler, Antoine Lutz, and Richard J Davidson.

2016. "Long-Term Mindfulness Training Is Associated with Reliable Differences in Resting Respiration Rate." *Psychophysiology.* doi:10.1038/srep27533.

Wilson, Annie. 2015. *How to Increase Gray Matters in the Brain.* Inner Light Publishers. http://www.inner-light-in.com/2015/01/how-to-increase-gray-matters-in-the-brain/.

Yang, Xiang, Da-chun Chen, Yun-long Tan, Shu-ping Tan, Zhi-ren Wang, Fu-de Yang, Olaoluwa O Okusaga, Giovana B Zunta-soares, and Jair C Soares. 2015. "The Interplay between BDNF and Oxidative Stress in Chronic Schizophrenia."

Zautra, Alex J., Robert Fasman, Mary C. Davis, and Arthur D (Bud) Craig. 2010. "The Effects of Slow Breathing on Affective Responses to Pain Stimuli: An Experimental Study." *Pain* 149 (1): 12–18. doi:10.1016/j.pain.2009.10.001.

www.ingramcontent.com/pod-product-compliance
Lightning Source LLC
Chambersburg PA
CBHW061438180526
45170CB00004B/1464